the
hot
belly
diet

the
hot
belly
diet

A 30-DAY AYURVEDIC PLAN TO RESET YOUR
METABOLISM, LOSE WEIGHT, AND RESTORE
YOUR BODY'S NATURAL BALANCE TO HEAL ITSELF

Dr. Suhas G. Kshirsagar
with Kristin Loberg

Foreword by Deepak Chopra, MD

ATRIA PAPERBACK

NEW YORK · LONDON · TORONTO · SYDNEY · NEW DELHI

ATRIA PAPERBACK

An Imprint of Simon & Schuster, Inc.
1230 Avenue of the Americas
New York, NY 10020

Copyright © 2014 by Dr. Suhas G. Kshirsagar

All rights reserved, including the right to reproduce this book or portions thereof in any form whatsoever. For information, address Atria Books Subsidiary Rights Department, 1230 Avenue of the Americas, New York, NY 10020.

First Atria Paperback edition December 2015

ATRIA PAPERBACK and colophon are trademarks of Simon & Schuster, Inc.

For information about special discounts for bulk purchases, please contact Simon & Schuster Special Sales at 1-866-506-1949 or business@simonandschuster.com.

The Simon & Schuster Speakers Bureau can bring authors to your live event. For more information or to book an event, contact the Simon & Schuster Speakers Bureau at 1-866-248-3049 or visit our website at www.simonspeakers.com.

Interior design by Paul Dippolito

Manufactured in the United States of America

10   9   8   7

Library of Congress Cataloging-in-Publication Data

Kshirsagar, Suhas G.
    The hot belly diet : a 30-day ayurvedic plan to reset your metabolism, lose weight, and restore your body's natural balance to heal itself / by Dr. Suhas G. Kshirsagar with Kristin Loberg ; foreword by Deepak Chopra.—First Atria Books hardcover edition.
        pages cm
    1. Weight loss. 2. Metabolism—Regulation. 3. Self-care, Health. I. Loberg, Kristin. II. Title.
    RM222.2.K796 2014
    613.2'5—dc23   2014003399

ISBN 978-1-4767-3480-4
ISBN 978-1-4767-3481-1 (pbk)
ISBN 978-1-4767-3482-8 (ebook)

*To all the people who wrestle with weight
and search for eternal well-being.*

*To those who have rekindled the fire in
their belly and illuminated their life.*

*And to my parents, who taught me patience, adaptability,
and resilience—the simple keys to a happy life.*

When diet is wrong, medicine is of no use.
When diet is correct, medicine is of no need.

—AYURVEDIC PROVERB

Contents

Contents

the
hot
belly
diet

Foreword

by Deepak Chopra, MD

Looking back, I find it astonishing to realize that almost everything that was left out of medical school training when I was becoming a physician now occupies center stage. I was taught nothing about the mind-body connection, which most of my professors would have scoffed at if it had been brought up. Thoughts and feelings were like ghosts in the machine, disconnected from the body. Prevention was considered unworthy of wasting time on—it could be left to hygienists and public health authorities. Nutrition was even low on the totem pole and could be left to home economics teachers in high school.

As for Eastern medical systems, they existed somewhere over the horizon, so far over that nothing about them was actually known before it could be dismissed. Now the situation has changed, and when I welcome *The Hot Belly Diet* as one of the most practical and useful ways to improve your life through Ayurveda, many readers will know what I'm referring to. Thanks to the popularity of integrative medicine, India's traditional system of Ayurveda—the term literally translates as "science of life"—has become another healing modality that is worthy of respect and study. More to the point, it has made invaluable contributions to self-care.

Self-care has become the dominant focus of prevention over the past few decades. In medical school, I was taught that health is the absence of disease, an entirely inadequate definition. Health is a positive state whose elements—balance, energy, a sense of well-being, resistance to disease, and the promoting of healing—are exactly what Ayurveda aims to maintain and nurture.

Dr. Suhas G. Kshirsagar has founded a thriving practice on his extensive knowledge of Ayurveda, so one would expect that his book contains a fund of fascinating information and guidance. At the same time, however, its basic principle is simple: The digestive tract is the most critical system in the body, because it supplies the energy that allows cells to go through their life cycle, from birth to death, in a state of perfect balance. The key concept is *agni*, the digestive fire, which supplies vitality to the whole mind-body system when it is burning brightly and efficiently. Moreover, the quality of your metabolism—the process of converting food energy into bodily tissues—decides the quality and quantity of the life you experience. If you have a humming metabolism fueled by *agni*, you will slow down your body's aging process and boost its overall health. This is the very basis of *The Hot Belly Diet*.

As used in India, agni crosses all kinds of boundaries. The original Sanskrit word can be literal (any fire is called "agni"), metaphorical (as in "digestive fire"), mythic (as in the sacrificial fires that ceremonially burn away evil and nourish good), and spiritual (the Vedic gods include one named Agni). This flagrant liberality would have appalled my medical-school professors, as proponents of Western scientific medicine (as was my father, one of the first British-trained cardiologists in postindependence India). But the need has since arisen to approach well-being from a holistic perspective. In reality, when mind and body are totally intertwined, respecting rigid boundaries makes little sense—in fact, it's bad medicine.

We are lucky to be living during an exciting time for self-care, prevention, and the rise of holistic health. More knowledge about health is available than ever before, yet society continues to suffer from serious lifestyle disorders that are largely preventable. Getting new MDs up to speed is still a problem, although integrative medicine is fast making inroads. So it's up to anyone who wants to maintain a high level of well-being to explore the possibilities personally. Dr. Kshirsagar is an excellent, reliable guide to the most important questions that we all face:

What is the wisdom of the body?

How can our innate healing system be supported?

What part does diet play in long-term health?

What is the best approach to slowing down and preventing the aging process?

There are mind-body answers to these questions, and since Ayurveda respected the wisdom of the body thousands of years before Western medicine stopped dismissing the concept out of hand, I think *The Hot Belly Diet* will prove invaluable.

A personal note: I first met Dr. Kshirsagar more than twenty years ago, during the height of the Transcendental Meditation movement, when I was just beginning to turn my focus to Ayurveda and mind-body medicine in general. I've seen him grow over the years as a compassionate healer and expert clinician who now directs Ayurvedic Healing, an integrative wellness clinic in Northern California. As a sought-after speaker and lecturer, he travels throughout the world teaching courses in Ayurveda, training doctors, and providing consultations for thousands of people.

In 2006 we started to work closely together, and he's become a regular teacher at The Chopra Center for Wellbeing, in Carlsbad, California, as well as a featured speaker at many of its signature programs and workshops. As one of my trusty advisers, he is responsible for helping me create a number of formulas and products rooted in our shared philosophy.

It's nice to see more people embracing the power of integrative medicine today, but many are still lost and confused—the things they've had drummed into them about prevention haven't turned into action. Change is hard. But as the obesity epidemic rages and lifestyle diseases remain the number one cause of fatality in America, people will keep wishing and hoping for the secret to perfect health. This book holds many such secrets. It will show you how to gain control over your waistline and guide you to the right way to eat for your body type (*dosha*) that current dieting fads cannot. May *The Hot Belly Diet* help you to bring mind-body balance, nourishment, and health into your life like never before. Dr. Kshirsagar has done all the hard work for you, telling you exactly what to do while also highlighting the pertinent science that he's diligently researched to make his ancient message come alive in the twenty-first century.

For all of these reasons, you need to turn to Ayurveda, and I can't think of a more qualified person than Dr. Kshirsagar to translate the concepts that I've been exploring and writing about for years into a practical program that anyone can access. The invitation is open; healing awaits.

PART ONE

Life

CHAPTER 1

Rekindle Your Fire, Rekindle Your Life

To eat is human, but to digest is divine.

—AYURVEDIC PROVERB

Jane was a forty-eight-year-old executive whose weight had crept up in recent years despite her constantly counting calories. When she came to see me, she was hoping I'd give her a secret formula for revving up her metabolism and effortlessly shedding the extra twenty pounds she'd been trying to lose to no avail. Her belly fat in particular bothered her the most, and it didn't budge even when she went to dieting extremes. She also wanted to gain back the vibrant energy that had escaped her some ten years ago, for she felt chronically tired, spent, and bloated. And she was clear with me that she knew everything there was to know about weight loss. While she admitted that she had no time to exercise during the week due to her constantly busy work at a large nonprofit, she followed all the other "rules" that stood at the center of virtually every popular diet of late: going low-carb; curbing refined sugars, gluten, dairy, and alcohol; making breakfast the most important meal of the day; and eating routinely throughout the day to dodge "dangerous" feelings of hunger.

But nothing was working. Her daily menu consisted of coffee for breakfast, a salad for lunch (dressing on the side), and whole wheat pasta for dinner with fish or chicken and a side of steamed vegetables. To prevent hunger pangs in between meals, she kept whole grain bars on hand. To say Jane was frustrated was an understatement. What probably surprised her the most was the question I asked her once she was done sharing with me her history and discontent: *Jane, I know you're here to seek help with your weight and low energy, but what is bugging you the most?*

Let's cut to the story of Macy for a moment, a forty-six-year-old African American woman who had struggled with her weight all her life. She had bloomed to 286 pounds when I first saw her in my office, and those last one hundred pounds had come on during the past decade. Macy was a teacher of nonviolent communication, but it was evident to me at our initial visit that, although she was an excellent listener with an intuitive sense of her students' inner thinking processes, Macy didn't listen to her own voice within. Her internal dialogue was as dead as her metabolism, and she wasn't connected to her own thoughts and body. Which is why she—like Jane—was taken aback by one of my first questions to her: *Macy, how do you feel in your body? What does it take for you to feel motivated?*

Now let's meet Craig, a twenty-nine-year-old CFO in Silicon Valley with high cholesterol and elevated blood sugar. About forty pounds overweight, he had no history of diabetes, but his blood work indicated that he was in a prediabetic state—a clear sign that his metabolism wasn't running efficiently and that his issues likely originated in his gut. His doctor wanted to put him on diabetes drugs and Lipitor, a popular cholesterol-lowering medication. Craig had previously visited me to deal with his acne, so he returned seeking help in taking control of his blood sugar and cholesterol without having to resort to drugs. And, like my other patients, Craig was bemused by my question to him: *Craig, what's going on in your life?*

Within a matter of weeks, I began to turn all three of these people's health around. Jane lost her first seven pounds by the three-week mark, and a total of sixteen pounds over the course of six weeks. That may not seem like a tremendous amount, compared to many people, but as her excess fat disappeared, including that stubborn belly fat, she gained precious muscle mass and recouped youthful energy. Macy's weight began to drop immediately and dramatically. Although when she first saw me she was afraid to go to the gym due to her weight, it didn't take long to get her motivated through our work together. When I explained to her that her life had become stagnant and sedentary and that this was reflective of her health and body, she agreed that she felt "trapped" and "boxed in" by her life's responsibilities and ongoing demands. Our goal, then, was to bring life, or *prana*, back into her so it could open up the channels of her body to support radiant health and ideal weight. And this task would start with her diet, which is how I launch all of my patients' transformations, since it immediately targets ground zero: the belly and how it metabolizes food to then give life and health to every other system in the body. Within just one week, Macy felt a huge difference in her level of energy and self-motivation. She also began to have positive conversations with herself that reinforced her confidence and good attitude. Over the first four weeks, she lost a whopping twenty-six pounds and was well on her way to achieving a goal weight that she'd never seen before in her entire life. She also began to experience a normal menstrual cycle, something she hadn't had in years. This was a true sign of her body returning to its natural, optimal state. With her metabolism made over and reset, everything else about her condition could follow a healing path to health.

For Craig, his remedy required that he pay attention to his job-related stress as we cleaned up his diet and rebooted his metabolism from the gut. It turned out that he'd been suffering extreme pressures both at work and at home, and I explained to him that the stress—more so than his food choices and lack of exercise—was what his body was responding to. No doctor had bothered to ask him what was going on in his life; they just wanted to prescribe chemicals that would mask the symptoms and leave the root of the problem untreated. In my view, Craig's liver, gallbladder, and pancreas—important collaborators with the belly in digesting food and managing the metabolism—were pissed off and angry. And, as you're about to learn, these organs are the seat of *agni,* a fiery life force in the body that drives and sustains wellness (not to mention ideal weight management). In addition to starting him on my dietary protocol, I encouraged him to meditate, to consider another job that wasn't so stressful, and to communicate better with his wife. This may seem like a tall order to fill, but it's not when you consider how Craig approached each objective I gave him that could fit within his lifestyle and current commitments.

Like so many of the people I treat, Jane, Craig, and Macy had all reached a point where they were literally scared to eat for fear of experiencing adverse effects to whatever they put in their mouth. They felt like something wasn't working in their belly, as if their ability to digest food had weakened no matter what they did to resolve the problem. And when I asked each of them to describe in words how they felt, the responses were similar: clogged, big, heavy, dull, and sleepy.

I know what you're asking: How exactly did these people turn their health around? What was their protocol? (In other words, what did they eat, avoid, do, and not do?) And what did my somewhat strange and unusual questions have to do with their cure?

Welcome to Ayurveda.

When people ask me to define Ayurveda, I begin by saying that it's a consciousness-based approach to health. Which then begs other questions, such as *What does that mean? How is Ayurveda really different from other alternative healing methods? Is there any proof to its effectiveness? What does Ayurveda have to do with weight loss?*

For starters, Ayurveda is one of the most ancient and comprehensive systems of health care that exist today. The term comes from the Sanskrit words *ayus* ("life") and *veda* ("knowledge"); it literally means "the knowledge or science of life." Ayurveda developed from the spiritual texts of ancient India called the *Vedas*, or "Books of Wisdom." These are at least five thousand years old and are widely revered as our oldest literature. And it's this very body of knowledge recorded long ago that's finally getting the recognition it deserves. Indeed, modern science now proves why an Ayurvedic approach to health can be so powerful and effective. While foremost offering a proven weight-loss program, *The Hot Belly Diet* teaches the principles of an Ayurvedic lifestyle through a highly practical and mainstream approach while rooting its lessons in the latest scientific research.

One of Ayurveda's core philosophies is the idea that within each and every one of us lies the capacity to live happy, balanced lives free of pain and disease. But to achieve this seemingly superhuman feat, we have to create the qualities of what's called "self-referral," which means you're connected to yourself in ways that allow you to optimize every aspect of yourself. In other words, you're able to effortlessly know and manage who you are, what your body type is, what your lifestyle choices should be, how to process emotions and stress, and how to interact with all the different fundamental qualities of nature around you while maintaining a semblance of balance. Granted, it's impossible to maintain balance at all times, and we all go through transitions in life that are normal, and expected. But having the awareness that you're constantly striving to do something good for your own mind, body, and spirit is the goal. And that's exactly what Ayurveda is all about. It's truly the science of life—the science of *experience*. Health, according to Ayurveda, is the ultimate byproduct of enlightenment. And, as this book will show, enlightenment can begin immediately with your diet.

I realize the idea that "enlightenment begins with diet" may sound like an absurd and abstract statement, but see if you can open yourself up to this new knowledge and experience what it can do for you. All that I ask at this juncture is that you choose health. That's the first step to take on the path to radiant wellness. It's what I made Jane, Macy, and Craig do during their first consultations with me. You can only be as healthy as you think possible. The second step, of course, is to reject the mentality that says disease is inevitable, or that "old age" implies illness and infirmity. I'm here to tell you emphatically that it does not.

Despite all that we know today in comparison to just one hundred years ago, disease still remains largely a mystery. Yes, we've decoded our DNA and created vaccines and antibiotics to combat known invaders. Yes, we've developed advanced diagnostic tools and sharpened our knives to revolutionize surgical techniques. But we still struggle mightily to deal with understanding why one person dies prematurely while another lives robustly for a long time. We've all heard of the athlete with no risk factors for coronary artery disease, yet who dies suddenly on the playing field of a heart attack; the lung cancer victim who never smoked; the skinny health nut who is diagnosed with diabetes or early-onset dementia; and the HIV-positive individual who never shows signs or symptoms of sickness and who never receives drugs or treatment. What explains these phenomena?

We may never know. I am reminded of (and amused by) a cartoon I once saw that depicted God deliberating over the fact we've decoded our DNA. He says something to the effect of, "Oh, no. I must change the password now."

I think we all can agree that in addition to accepting a certain mystery surrounding the body's functionality, and whether or not it becomes sick and enfeebled, how we choose to live—and think—has a profound effect on our health and psychology. It's far easier, and cheaper, to prevent illness than to treat it once it's established. And prevention cannot happen the way treatments are often delivered—targeted to one specific area. There is no such thing as "spot prevention"; we have to honor the body as a whole, complex unit. This is why Ayurveda can be so powerful. It tells us that the mind exerts the greatest influence on the body, and avoiding sickness demands that we bring our own awareness into balance and extend that balance to the body. This in turn manifests in a higher state of health.

The Doctor Is In

Before I get to the details of what you can expect from this diet, let me introduce myself. The journey I have taken over the past twenty-plus years will give you a sense of how I've created this program and why I am so thrilled to share it with you, given the results I've seen among my own patients.

If you haven't figured it out by now, I am not a traditional Western doctor with an American degree. And I do things differently in my office. I was born in India. My early years were very typical of a young Indian boy born into a family of Brahmans—the "custodians of Vedic culture"—who are obligated to follow Ayurvedic scripture. *Brahman* refers to a certain class of people in traditional Hindu societies who, because of their lineage, are responsible for becoming the spiritual leaders and healers in a noble profession. So, in a sense, I was destined to become a doctor and teacher; in fact, at the age of eight I was officially initiated into this duty and went on to spend the next two decades participating in rigorous study with various authorities and gurus, including distinguished physicians and scholars from all over the world. My journey has been a remarkable one. After interacting with vastly different health-care communities, schools of thought, cultures, and methods of practice around the globe, I've integrated what I've seen and experienced into a unique set of skills rooted in my Ayurvedic foundation.

Food and herbal formulations have always been at the heart of my practice. During my formal training, I learned that food was equally as important in the healing process as the medicine itself. The hospitals where I worked were equipped with elaborate kitchens, and that's where I was taught how to design special foods for patients as well as give special importance to where the problem was coming from—rather than just acknowledge the symptoms.

I earned my Bachelor of Ayurvedic Medicine and Surgery (BAMS) from Pune University in its namesake city southeast of Mumbai, then continued onward with my education to gain an MD in Ayurvedic medicine from Pune. Following graduation, I started to practice medicine in a rural area on the outskirts of Pune until, one day, Maharishi Mahesh Yogi, the father of the Transcendental Meditation movement, invited me to join his team in Holland. This would change everything in my life, for Maharishi was seeking traditional Ayurvedic physicians to bring Ayurveda to the West. I was twenty-five years old at the time and skeptical about teaching Ayurveda outside my Eastern culture. But I made a leap of faith, moved, and never looked back. I traveled to thirty-eight countries during my ten years with Maharishi, eventually landing in America in 1999 to direct the world-famous Panchakarma health center in Fairfield, Iowa. While based in Fairfield, I continued to travel extensively throughout the United States to teach.

Entering Western culture had a profound impact on me. Aside from learning English, the immersion into a Western way of life gave me a new perspective about the world and my role in it. It didn't take long for me to notice the far-reaching effects that the Western diet was having on many people, which I saw as lacking in essential nutrients. My Ayurvedic background had taught me that food was medicine, but I wasn't seeing "medicinal" meals anywhere. This motivated me to find ways to nourish my patients by providing them with simple, practical cooking secrets that would result in meals that contained all the building blocks of the body and were easy to digest and prepare. They also had to meet two other high standards: (1) have a rejuvenating detox effect, and (2) have a calming effect on the mind, since so many of my patients were fighting daily stress and anxiety. Soon enough, I started recommending the ancient recipes of my Indian upbringing to my patients, and the results I was witnessing spoke for themselves.

I counsel an enormous array of people from all walks of life, many of whom visit me at my clinic in Santa Cruz once they've exhausted traditional Western medicine's approach to treating certain conditions, or who just want to "feel better" following a long bout with vague, undiagnosed symptoms. Some hope to reduce their vulnerability to future illness and disease, while at the same time learn new strategies for coping with stress, tension, and worry, and achieve a more stable emotional state. I am very up front with my patients from the moment I meet them. I clearly ask them what their objective is, and I probe deeply into their lifestyle and dietary habits like few other traditional doctors do during initial consults. In addition to routine questions about their medical history, medications, supplements, and chief concerns, I ask about their spiritual practices, work, sex life, levels of stress, ability to make decisions, quality of sleep, type of nighttime dreams, and vulnerability to things like jealousy, envy, rage, and over-attachment. I even go so far as to inquire about which tastes they prefer, what time of day they eat their meals, how they plan their days, and whether or not they are experiencing stress in any close relationship.

As I did with Jane, Macy, and Craig, my first questions often seem unrelated to their complaints or reasons for being in my office, but no sooner do I ask people what's bothering them the most than the truth comes out. And the "truth" is often at the heart of their health and weight struggles. Most of the time, it's not about the weight per se. Indeed, they are well aware of the extra weight, but what's troubling them more than anything are all of the symptoms they have for which traditional medicine cannot seem to remedy quickly. Once I put them on my plan, however, their organs and organ systems start regulating themselves. They start to feel a flow of energy they've never felt before. The weight starts to disappear. And so do their myriad symptoms.

Over the past two decades, I've treated more than fifteen thousand patients and trained thousands of other health-care providers in Ayurvedic theory and practice. I've also collaborated with prominent physicians to design treatment protocols and formulate new health and wellness programs and products. At the Chopra Center, for instance, I train its staff and medical doctors to acquire the language and tools needed to incorporate an Ayurvedic approach into its practice. A classic example of this would be a case whereby a patient is complaining of insomnia. In addition to identifying any underlying medical causes for the condition, I help determine what kind of imbalance in the body could be causing the trouble. If the person has trouble falling asleep, it's likely the sign of a *vata* imbalance; if he or she falls asleep fine, but then wakes up later in the night with a racing mind, unable to go back to sleep, then a *pitta* imbalance is likely to blame; and if the individual has a hard time waking up in the morning and getting started with lots of natural energy, then I'd point to a *kapha* imbalance. If these terms—vata, pitta, kapha—are foreign to you, hang tight. You will soon come to understand what they mean, and how they each relate to you. I am going to help you better understand your body and its inherent preferences and proclivities. This will allow you to finally find a lifelong plan of action you can sustain that will support your well-being (and your ideal waistline!).

To be clear, Ayurveda is not a substitute for traditional Western medicine. It expands our knowledge and adds a necessary dimension to conventional training. Blending Ayurveda with Western science brings together two sets of wisdom that work in brilliant synchronicity and have proven to be compatible. Contrary to popular belief, I am not one who depends solely on what some would call naturopathic remedies. Indeed, my practice honors the curative power of herbs, spices, and foods, but I also have a deep respect for how Western doctors practice, and I work side by side with them every day, relying on the same objective tests to understand a person's health status. But what I do in addition, that many conventional doctors do not, is guide patients to look inward and to find that all-important balanced awareness within themselves. I teach them how to honor their body's own intelligence, which is more powerful than any of us can imagine. This is what sets me apart.

I've learned that if I can convince people to do something for two weeks, I can change them for a lifetime. Over the course of my practice in America, I began to create a unique protocol for my patients that could address a broad spectrum of problems yet have just one simple formula: food filled with life and the tools to know how to find what works for each of them to maintain a humming digestive fire. This has evolved into the diet plan that's in this book and that you can now benefit from.

The Hot Belly Diet in Brief

The Hot Belly Diet is a rallying cry for anyone who hasn't been able to lose weight permanently and discover true health. Why a diet from an Ayurvedic point of view? Because I'm a firm believer that all roads to perfect health—and an ideal weight—begin with your mind-set, and your diet is the most important factor in creating that mentality. Food is information, after all; it gives your body the fuel it needs to survive (and, ideally, thrive) and helps generate the connection between what you think and do, and how you feel. What you eat directly impacts how you experience life and nourish your body's needs all the way down to your waistline. And this, my friends, is the essence of Ayurveda. By trying my 30-day protocol described in this book, you will experience this for yourself.

More and more, I treat people who've tried everything to reclaim the health that they deserve and who fall victim to fad diets and questionable health practices that seriously compromise their physical well-being. The laments I hear daily are constant: low energy, body-weight chaos, digestive disorders, poor sleep, headaches, congestion, low libido, low-grade depression, anxiety, burnout, and signs of ongoing inflammation such as sore joints or relentless allergies. The irony in all this is that many of these people are indeed active—they lead healthy lifestyles and yet fail to experience optimal health. Well, the reason is that these myriad conditions actually have a surprising common denominator: a weak digestive "fire." If you don't keep your digestive fires burning cleanly, you cannot lose weight permanently or achieve the vibrant health you've always dreamed of. What exactly do I mean by this? You'll get those details in the next chapter. But let me offer a primer here.

In Ayurveda, a healthy digestive system is seen as a cornerstone of well-being; as such, disease and disorder are believed to arise from inefficient digestion. In fact, we can even distill the science of Ayurveda down to the simple idea that total health resides in the state of our digestive powers, and that restoring health must originate with a focus on our digestive system. Your digestive fire simply refers to your body's metabolism—the process of turning nutrients from food into energy for cells to sustain life, which, of course, is commandeered by your digestion, a complex combination of biological and chemical interactions. And the ingredients that make for a strong digestion and fast metabolism or "fire" include four chief components:

1. Eating specific foods and drinking certain hot liquids that feed and fuel your metabolism rather than slow it down, ultimately supporting digestive balance and efficiency. We know that, scientifically speaking, not all calories are created equal. When you consume calories from the types of foods on the Hot Belly Diet, you can spur rapid weight loss. What's more, when you drink warm teas and water throughout the day, you can continually stoke your metabolism.

2. Fasting in between meals (no snacking), for the sensation of hunger is essential to weight loss and overall health. New sci-

ence shows that intermittent fasting can help you live a longer, healthier life.

3. Making lunch the most important meal of the day (i.e., eating when the sun is burning brightest). Studies now prove that eating more calories midday can result in greater weight loss, and that late lunches and big dinners can be detrimental to weight-loss efforts and general health—even if the total calories consumed in a day are the same.

4. Clearing out "digestive sludge"—residue from poorly digested food that antagonizes weight loss, provokes hormonal imbalances, and ultimately triggers inflammation, the root cause of virtually all disease. This sludge also includes toxins that cannot be cleared by the body effectively due to a weak metabolism and debilitated digestive organs such as the pancreas and liver. Research now shows that these toxins, which are created by the body during normal metabolism, can trigger weight gain and impede weight-loss efforts. Removing this sludge, however, is like clearing dust and ashes from a used fireplace to get the logs to burn stronger and cleaner the next time. You'll achieve this through a combination of steps in addition to the diet, including a twenty-four-hour castor oil cleanse, healing waters (i.e., herbal teas), and some herbal supplements you can take that are widely available today.

At the core of this four-part, three-phase diet is a dish called *khichadi* (pronounced kitch-a-dee)—a complete but incredibly easy-to-make meal that helps clear out that digestive sludge and transform your metabolism. Overall, the Hot Belly Diet changes your relationship with food to make healthy eating—and living—effortless.

I want to emphasize that this isn't another diet that severely restricts your calories and has an unrealistic "Do Not Eat" column to abide by. I won't tell you to go totally gluten free or low carb. True, gluten-free diets help some people to a certain extent.

But the vast majority of us just need to reprogram how we think about the foods we eat, how we prepare them in combination with other foods, and when we choose to eat them. You'll be rejoicing at the fact that this diet is based on carbohydrates, showing you how to use carbs smartly to feel lighter and purer in body, mind, and spirit. Anyone who has twisted their own arm in a bid to go low-carb forever knows what an impossible feat that can be. And it's wholly unnatural, as you're about to find out from both an Ayurvedic and a scientific standpoint. We know now that the body needs carbohydrates like it needs air and water. We also know that vibrant health isn't about the hours spent on a treadmill and eating a balanced breakfast. In fact, I'll make a case for skipping breakfast entirely and explain why it could be the ticket to rapid, healthy weight loss. More than anything, the Hot Belly Diet is about how your meals are digested to either fuel your fire of health or dampen it. And this is a simple reflection of which types of foods we eat at which times of day.

I trust that most of you will start to feel the effects of this diet within a matter of days. But it will take a full month for it to have a lasting impact on your body at both the cellular and metabolic levels. It also takes that long to reset your mentality so that you can effortlessly enjoy a new lifestyle.

So here's the Hot Belly Diet at a glance:

The Quick and Easy Overview of the Hot Belly Diet

Phase ❶ Prepare: Days 1–3

Starting with an optional castor oil cleanse on the first day, this brief phase begins to detox the body, kills cravings, and starts to rev that metabolic engine—that hot belly fire. You'll learn several key dietary dos and don'ts during this phase and train your mind and body to think differently when it comes to food. You'll also be simultaneously training your tongue to taste differently as you cut out sugar, meat, processed carbs, artificial sweeteners, and full-fat dairy. You'll be less swayed by cravings and the urge to overeat. This is when "kindling" is being introduced, a metaphor for the physical shift in your body's biology whereby digestive powers are beginning to be renovated and turned on maximally for optimal digestion.

Phase ❷ Accelerate: Days 4–26

During this 21-day segment, you'll follow a specific protocol that's laid out for you meal by meal, day by day—with all simple and portable recipes provided. It entails a protein shake in the morning, a bowl of khichadi at lunch and dinner (with the lunch version bigger than the dinner one), and fasting in between meals to maximally stoke your fire and not inhibit fat-burning. Even the most time-starved and "on-the-go" reader will find this phase doable and effortless. A few optional ideas are offered for lunch, which is the most important meal of the day. The purpose of Phase 2 is to set the stage for you to reintroduce foods after three weeks and welcome a leaner, happier you. In Ayurvedic medicine, the secrets to metabolic acceleration encompass *deepana,* which means "bioactivator," and *pachana,* which means "bioaccelerator." As these words suggest, the goal is to stimulate appetite and prepare digestion to extract nutrients quickly and easily once food arrives.

Phase ❸ Transform: Days 27–30 and Beyond

These four days are used to teach you how to keep the weight loss going while also reintroducing certain foods back into your diet. A final cleanse on the last day is optional. What you'll learn in this phase sets you up for a lifetime of enjoying a healthy digestive fire.

You'll be asked to incorporate as many of the twenty-one tips outlined in Chapter 9 as you can, if you haven't already!

■ ■ ■

Truth be told, this diet will allow you to shed eight to ten pounds quickly, within 30 days. Many people, however, will lose considerably more depending on their unique conditions and commitment to the plan. You will continue to lose weight after the 30 days using my guidelines. I'll be going into all the details of the diet in the upcoming chapters, but as a very quick summary, the Hot Belly Diet is a delicious, easy, and enlightening way to establish a new relationship not only with food and eating, but with yourself. Even if you're among the lucky few who don't have a lot of weight to lose and who aren't currently diagnosed with a serious condition, this program can still have profoundly transformative effects on your sense of well-being and your future health.

One thing I want you to keep in mind from the get-go is that often people who try to lose weight ultimately fail because they are bullied by undeniable cravings and a false sense of hunger, both of which are really just reflections of unfulfilled desires that can be satisfied beyond food. When you crave a snack, for example, what you're really craving is something sweet or salty, but not necessarily food per se to satisfy true hunger. In other words, your body might not be hungry at all in terms of needing energy, yet your tongue wants to taste something (which is why most snacks are loaded with sugar, salt, and often fat). But many times that "craving" can be killed with plain water or a social distraction like talking to a good friend (indeed, false hunger can also be the result of pure boredom). Throughout this book, I'm going to reiterate the importance of learning how to differentiate between real and fake hunger. Is your belly hungry? Or just your tongue and inner psyche?

Once I'm done teaching you the basics of this diet and how to follow it, I will then spend time sharing how to maximize and maintain this new way of life. We need to rise above the idea that food is the only thing that provides nourishment. In Ayurveda, nourishment comes from everything and everywhere—the air, the soil, the water, our relationships, and so on.

Do we need to become sick and grow old at all? People have asked this question for centuries. According to Ayurvedic wisdom, if the digestive forces inside us are correctly balanced with the surrounding environment, we can be immune to illness. Perfect balance makes perfect health possible. And that's exactly the premise from which the Hot Belly Diet is born.

I'm excited to get you started, so without further ado, let's begin with an understanding of how you're going to return life to your body with life from food. Part of this lesson entails busting pervasive myths that circle the diet world today, and another part involves your figuring out through a few fun and simple quizzes which type of digestive fire you have, so you can then maximize all the rewards of the Hot Belly Diet. I know you can do this. It doesn't matter how often you've failed following diets in the past or how much doubt you have in the effectiveness of Ayurveda. What matters is that you focus on your goals and have faith that health and happiness await you.

CHAPTER 2

Cracking the Ancient Code to Vibrant Health

The body is the outcome of food. Even so, disease is the outcome of food. The distinction between ease and disease arises on account of wholesome nutrition or the lack of it, respectively.

—CHARAKA, ONE OF THE PRINCIPAL CONTRIBUTORS TO THE ANCIENT ART AND SCIENCE OF AYURVEDA; BORN IN 300 BC, HE IS REFERRED TO AS THE FATHER OF MEDICINE

If I had to sum up the Hot Belly Diet in two words, it would be this: digestive fire. Now, this may seem like an incredibly esoteric or "new age" concept, but it's one of the oldest ideas on the planet, and one that modern science can prove with astonishing implications for anyone who wants to live a long, lean life. The Hot Belly Diet is a revolutionary diet plan grounded in today's science, but it combines several different strategies rooted in the ancient science of Ayurveda to help you do more than just lose inches around your waist. You'll experience a transformation in your overall wellness, level of contentment, and confidence. Although you may have come to this book with singular hopes of watching the scale tick downward as the pounds drop off, I want you to set your sights higher than that as you simultaneously reduce your risk for many illnesses and conditions and feel your energy and enthusiasm for life soar. I think it's quite telling, in fact, that one of the oldest words in modern science, dating back to the late seventeenth century, is *eupeptic,* which means having good digestion and being cheerful and optimistic. The two—healthy digestion and happiness—go hand in hand. (It's no wonder that general good health and a sense of well-being hinge on the state of your digestion, for your gastrointestinal tract is the largest and arguably most important part of your immune system, as you'll soon understand.)

The core Accelerate Phase of the Hot Belly Diet is extremely simple and straightforward and can be customized to meet any dietary preference, but at the same time, it's designed to limit the flexibility that can derail a dieter and to allow for maximum results that put you on a path to a lifetime of healthy eating habits. The Hot Belly Diet spells out in detail each meal you will eat during the Accelerate Phase, but it also gives you some wiggle room to make substitutions so that you can swap some ingredients and even entire meals if you like.

Although I will ask you to refrain from eating certain foods during the Accelerate Phase, this isn't because I believe them to be "bad" or "unhealthy." Many of today's diets demonize particular ingredients like gluten, dairy, meat, alcohol, caffeine, and nonorganic anything, but they do so for the wrong reasons. Granted, some people have issues with these ingredients and would do well to stay away from them. But from my perspective, the problem rests in cherry-picking nutrition. I have worked with so many individuals who have tried these elimination diets to no avail. Indeed, they lose weight initially, but then they either cannot keep the weight loss going or revert back to old habits, and the weight comes surging back on. Moreover, they don't typically feel good as they uncomfortably force themselves to avoid the foods they've come to love and aim to follow a strict, sometimes expensive protocol.

The other problem with cherry-picking nutrition is that it can lead to unintended consequences. If high-fiber, whole grain pancakes, for instance, are deemed "good," then you can find yourself piling on other "good" things like nuts, fruit, and real maple syrup until it becomes a very heavy, dense meal that sabotages your efforts to lose weight. Just because it's healthy and organic (and free of "bad" ingredients) doesn't make it good for you and your waistline. Another example I encounter frequently is filling in nutritional blanks with synthetics (i.e., mega-dosing on vitamins and capsules marketed as substitutes for fruits and vegetables). Few people understand that popping a pill is not the same as eating authentic whole food; isolated nutritional compounds that are swallowed are not assimilated well into the body, and they give people a false sense of security. What's more, taking such synthetics can wreak havoc on existing conditions, not to mention weaken liver function. I've had patients, for instance, who are already taking blood pressure medication and who also take synthetic calcium pills in a bid to boost their calcium levels and "protect their bones." These calcium supplements, however, have an effect whereby they trigger hardening of not just bone, but other areas of the body such as the blood vessels (which, in turn, increases blood pressure!). I have to tell these people that they need to get their calcium from the right source. And no sooner do they lighten up on their calcium intake and switch to natural sources of calcium than they watch their levels normalize. This theme has played out in numerous other cases I've encountered—people who don't realize that these concentrated XYZ pills are backing up their liver, slowing down their digestion, and creating an overall sluggish intestinal and metabolic environment that conflicts with their health and weight goals.

My whole point in bringing up these examples is to show you how it's virtually impossible to selectively choose one or a few things to portray as wicked and formulate an entire diet around that. It's also difficult to focus solely on what you eat when you're trying to lose weight permanently. There are just so many other things that factor into one's overall weight and whether or not losing extra pounds is relatively effortless or requires a Herculean effort. Which is why the Hot Belly Diet is decidedly different. The Hot Belly Diet is about eating whole foods that have been known to mankind for centuries and that don't confuse the body or slow its metabolic processes. It's also about eating at particular times during the day when your digestion is strongest, and letting hunger build in between meals. I'll also be equipping you with additional (un-diet-related) strategies that will enhance your ability to gain control of your waistline once and for all. You may not think, for example, that how you perceive yourself and what you do to take care of your psyche and self-motivation have any direct effect on how many calories you can burn or what your blood pressure is, but understanding your general life's circumstances and the challenges you face—including ones that have nothing to do with your weight—plays powerfully into the size of your waistline. This is exactly what Ayurveda has to offer: a new lens through which you can understand yourself and what will work for you in terms of losing weight, keeping it off, and gaining radiant health. After all, we don't say "She has a fire in her belly" for nothing. We all need an element of fire within us to be healthy and happy . . . and to even pursue the goal of getting healthier. Fire is positively symbolic in so many ways. And it also correlates with a healthy burning desire for certain things in life that make us fulfilled.

I think we all can agree that life is about so much more than our weight and dietary choices; and it extends far beyond mere chronological age or even physical health. This is how Ayurveda sees it, too. "Life," or ayus, is a fusion of the mind, body, senses, and soul. As such, Ayurveda respects the nature of life through the lens of Mother Nature herself. It shows us how to be compatible with the basic laws of nature, offering a road map for acknowledging and awakening our own inherent healing potential. The fundamental principle of Ayurvedic medicine is simple and empowering: You can become your own best doctor if you acknowledge the power of self-healing.

Ayurveda also teaches that health cannot be defined by lab tests or annual check-ups (nor the number on the scale and your cholesterol level!). There is no such thing as an "average person" or "one-size-fits-all" standard treatment. Much to the contrary, health is a continuous process that demands constant participation and embraces all aspects of "life"—from the physical, mental, and emotional, to the behavioral, spiritual, social, and so on. True health is the achievement of balance in all aspects, and each one of us is unique and requires a special, distinct blueprint for health. This explains why each one of us can respond so differently to various treatments, drugs, and dietary protocols. That said, Ayurveda does provide a general foundation for honoring all of these blueprints. It shows us how to acknowledge and support our true individual natures. Likewise, the Hot Belly Diet offers you the blueprint for understanding your own inner metabolic constitution for achieving optimal health and weight maintenance.

I realize that many of you have likely tried other diets before, and you look toward this book seeking yet another "solution." With so many programs available, it's a legitimate question: Why would you choose this one over another? The answer lies in the words I employed to sum up the diet at the beginning: digestive fire. When you come to understand what digestive fire—*hot belly*—means, and what a focus on this little-known aspect of healthy physiology can do for you, you'll soon know exactly why the road to wellness and ideal weight hinges on it (and why other diets might have failed you). The majority of people who have tried the early version of this diet repeatedly share that unlike other plans they have tried, they could see themselves following this one forever. It makes sense to them, and perhaps more important, it makes sense to their bodies, too.

Time to Ignite Your Digestive Fire

Before I get to the technical definition of digestive fire, let's briefly return to the people you met a few pages ago in Chapter 1. This will give you a sense of how Ayurveda shapes this diet and how it relates to the idea of digestive fire.

First, we had Jane, who was eating a lot of processed, packaged foods in the name of diet, such as energy bars, gluten-free products, and sugar-free items. She was also replacing real meat with fake meat (again, in the name of "diet"). Getting protein in the form of soy protein isolate, for instance, isn't the same as consuming proteins through whole foods such as fish and quinoa. Jane said that her body felt "yucky," and once I pointed out that the quality of her food would create the body that she wanted, she soon saw how her erroneous thinking about "diet foods" had led her astray. And she began to respect a relationship between the quality of her thinking and the state of her body.

Macy, on the other hand, was fooling herself as she motivated others in her daily work while feeling wholly unmotivated herself. She wasn't walking her talk, and the negativity she felt toward herself and her body was creating emotional blockages that manifested in physical conditions such as panic attacks and even heart palpitations. She had nothing to look forward to in her life, and a halo of sadness hovered over her. None of this, of course, helped her make good nutritional choices as her weight ballooned to nearly 290 pounds. Once I brought to her attention that it's easy to be "two-faced"—to do one thing at work and another at home—she could identify the disconnect and take action. At this writing, Macy's weight is at 168 pounds, and her goal is 150. I know she'll get there.

And then we had Craig, who also suffered a serious disconnect between his mind and body. He was young, but he was burned out from his job. He was performing more mental work than physical work and had to find a balance, or his body would continue to negatively react to everything going on in his stressful life. Just a little awareness of this misalignment was enough to set him on the right track back to health.

Despite each of these individuals' personal challenges, they shared a lot in common. All three of them lacked a strong connection with their bodies that could then inform their dietary and general lifestyle choices. This created an imbalance reflected by their weight struggles. And for someone like me, an Ayurvedic doctor who looks at the whole person rather than a small, isolated segment, my first order of business is to understand the root cause of a person's struggles that makes them overweight. Rarely is it a problem with a commonplace ingredient like wheat, or too many doughnuts. I often need to dig much deeper and look at what's driving a person's motivation to choose an unhealthy lifestyle. How did they drift away? When did they become less inspired? What threw their bodies off balance and how can we get them back into equilibrium? Which body type do they possess and how can I return it to that place where it functions in terrific coordination with their environment?

According to Ayurveda, your mind-body constitution, or dosha, is determined the moment you are conceived and your unique combination of the vata, pitta, and kapha doshas remains the same for life. In Sanskrit we call this *prakruti*, which simply means "nature."

Your prakruti is your foundation or base point. It dictates what keeps you in synch with your nature and thus healthy, and what can cause you to become imbalanced and sick (and overweight or obese). And you can't change your prakruti just as you can't change your genetically determined height and natural eye color.

Conversely, *vikruti* refers to a person's current state of imbalanced doshas. When I first consult with people, I focus on their vikruti rather than prakruti, as this will tell me what underlying imbalances need to be addressed. This is why I asked Jane, Macy, and Craig questions about the goings-on in their life and how they felt from a psychological standpoint before asking anything about weight-related matters. In Ayurveda, the essence of excellent health revolves around maintaining balance in the body and mind, which entails living in tune with one's personal mind-body constitution. And by evaluating an individual's vikruti, I can gather vital information about what kinds of shifts in lifestyle are required to return the body to a state of balance and well-being. In the next chapter,

I'll describe these doshas in greater detail and give you a way to determine which dosha dominates in you so you can learn more about your vikruti as you proceed.

So how does the concept of digestive fire fit in? As you can rightfully guess by now, the Hot Belly Diet isn't just a diet. I'm going to give you a revolutionary way of looking at the body and its rhythms that drive it either toward or away from ideal weight and health. Digestive fire and, conversely, intestinal sludge are probably concepts you've never heard of before, but once understood, these will change your weight-loss experience—your entire approach to health—for life.

Second to your individual dosha and current doshic state, agni is the most essential factor in governing your dietary needs. Agni, or the "digestive fire," is one of the most important, core principles in Ayurveda. Broadly speaking, it refers to your ability to process all aspects of life, including tangible things like food and drink to memories and even sensorial experiences. More specifically, your digestive fire, or agni, is the collection of digestive processes that are required to convert food into high-quality tissues and energy for cells. And those processes involve all the digestive juices, hormonal secretions, enzymes, and the activity that are needed to get the body's cylinders firing. (In fact, the words *ignite* and *ignition* come from the Sanskrit word agni. There are in fact a total of thirteen different agnis presiding over our metabolic functions. Any biochemical process or reaction in the body relates to agni. And in the bigger picture, agni is viewed as the creative force of intelligence that resides in all life.)

If we were to use more modern, technical terms, we'd say that your digestive fire is simply the body's fund of digestive enzymes, acids, biochemicals, hormones, and other substances it needs to properly metabolize foods so they can be broken down into usable parts, transported into destination cells, and carried to various areas of the body to conduct chores essential to keeping you alive. It's located within the lower stomach and small intestine, but finds its way throughout the entire body to preside over life-sustaining processes.

Although agni literally means fire, in the body it can be compared to your metabolism. It's responsible for absorbing the essential nutrients the body needs while getting rid of waste products. And if this critical part is functioning effectively, the whole body will be nourished, full of life and vitality. If our agni is strong, we build healthy appetites, and digest food efficiently. Agni gives our organs the strength to work optimally, and our minds emotional stability, clarity, and resilience.

> *Ayurveda identifies four main states of agni: balanced, irregular, sharp, and weak. When our agni is balanced, it ensures proper nourishment, energy levels, regular elimination, strong immunity, a clear complexion, excellent circulation, and overall strength and vitality.*

On the other hand, if our agni is weak, we can't digest efficiently, creating toxic residue, or *ama,* that gets trapped in our bodies. Ama is considered the root cause of disease. And its accumulation leads to a slow deterioration of the body. It also incapacitates our ability to process emotions, which in turn creates more toxic residue. For this reason, repressed anger, ongoing sadness, and chronic guilt are often seen in Ayurveda as being more debilitating than problems with physical digestion.

So contrary to what you might initially have thought, a hot digestive fire burning bright in your belly isn't solely about metabolism and it isn't just about digestion, either (and it's clearly not about heartburn!). It's about maintaining the body's overall *homeostasis*—the body's preferred state of being, a perfect balance whereby hor-

Agni and Ama

Agni and ama have contrasting properties. Agni is hot, dry, light, clear, and aromatic. It can metaphorically refer to the fire within a wood-burning stove. Ama, on the other hand, is cold, wet, heavy, cloudy, and foul-smelling. It's like the black build-up of soot in a chimney. The cleaner and more efficiently the wood burns, the more heat (energy) is produced, and the less toxins are created. This metaphor is emblematic of what happens in our digestive system, depending on its health. To treat ama, it is necessary to increase agni.

Signs of Healthy Agni
- Vibrant energy
- Clear, glowing skin
- Mental clarity
- Brightness in the eyes
- Sensation of hunger for next meal
- Regular bowel movements
- Well-formed stools

mones and other biomolecules are flowing as they should. It's about ridding the body of toxins that slow down its vital systems and clog its natural drains, and it's about gaining control of ama. If the sweet nectars of the body are water and blood, then ama is the gunk that impairs our ability to digest food. Undigested and partially digested food lingers, leading to the formation of this intestinal sludge that plugs up not only the intestines, but also other vital pathways, such as blood vessels and the movement of hormones in the body. As ama undergoes a multitude of chemical changes that wind up creating toxins in the bloodstream, it ultimately allows these toxins to accumulate in the weaker parts of the body, where they disrupt organs and cripple the immune system's powers. Eventually the end result is a disease state, which can manifest as heart disease, cancer, or an autoimmune disorder, among other ailments.

Ama is one of the most menacing barriers to good health. And here's the problem with virtually all diet systems currently on the market: They focus on calorie restriction through foods that merely perpetuate this intestinal swampland—causing serious buildup on our insides that antagonizes weight maintenance and can even lead to conditions such as irritable bowel syndrome, food allergies, celiac disease, and, as I just mentioned, cancer. The statistics tell the story: As we've witnessed a radical shift in the quality of our food supply coupled with our "toxic hunger" for anemic food found in processed and packaged products, we've simultaneously witnessed a dramatic increase in chronic conditions and diseases that can be linked back to this notion of ama.

> *Is my digestive fire weak? Quick test: The hallmark sign of weak digestion is* postprandial narcosis. *If you feel sleepy after eating a meal, it means you have very weak digestion. You have thrown a log on a very weak fire and blocked your essential system of energy extraction, so you feel like dozing off for an hour or two.*

I realize that I'm not using scientific terms that you're probably used to reading about in the media or modern health journals, but we can easily translate this philosophy to today's vocabulary. The body contains many types of agni. In your digestive system, for example, agni determines the production of hydrochloric acid in the stomach and sugar-digesting enzymes in the pancreas. It also regulates the thyroid gland and the metabolic changes in tissues from various signals in the body. Each cell has special agnis that work at a molecular level. So we can say that the metabolic pathway of agni begins with digestion and ends in the cells. Another way of looking at ama is to consider it the residual, poorly digested food particles like undigested proteins, excess sugars, and fats that get into the bloodstream and wreak metabolic havoc, triggering hormonal disturbances such as blood-sugar imbalances, insulin resistance, and, at the extreme, diabetes and other serious conditions. It can be recognized today as high cholesterol, hypertension, and digestive disorders such as acute constipation and/or diarrhea, among other health challenges. Although there is no equivalent in Western medicine to ama, it's well documented and widely accepted that toxins typically originate in the digestive tract. While some toxins, called *exogenous* toxins, can enter our body directly from the foods we eat (e.g., pesticides, herbicides, and antibiotic-treated meat and poultry), most are *endogenous*—a normal outcome of our body's digestive and metabolic processes as we turn nutrients from food into energy for cellular life. But if any of these toxins are not properly dealt with and neutralized, they can be harmful. Ama first accumulates in the colon and small intestine and then travels throughout the body via the blood. Put simply, ama creates toxic breeding grounds and acts as a precursor to disease.

In Ayurvedic thinking, all diseased states stem from ama, whether physical or mental, and ama is always the result of an improperly functioning agni. Ama pushes the body's underlying constitution into a state of disharmony. In a state of balance, on the other hand, the body removes ama with its own self-cleansing mechanisms through the bladder, bowels, lungs (i.e., breathing), and skin (i.e., sweat glands). In fact, the key to a healthy agni is the soul of the Hot Belly Diet: the consumption of fresh, easily digestible, compatible foods eaten consciously at the appropriate times. And that's what this diet teaches. Moreover, it helps you to cater to your unique agni.

We all know that each one of us digests food differently. You may radiate with satisfaction and a happy belly after a meal that irritates another person's digestion. As we'll see in upcoming chapters, we can turn to the doshas to help explain such disparities. We can also look at dosha-specific ways to reduce ama and encourage the body's natural cleansing mechanisms. Balanced pitta individuals, for example, enjoy an inherent fiery nature that helps them to break down and assimilate food into their bodies. So they are less likely to experience digestive problems (and be said to have an "iron stomach"). But this same person can suffer from an agni that's too strong and that can cause hyperacidity, heartburn, acid reflux, diarrhea, and excessive hunger. Similarly, the kapha-imbalanced person can harbor a weak agni that manifests in slow digestion, obesity, hypertension, diabetes, excess mucus, coughing, loss of appetite, and lethargy.

People who suffer from autoimmune disorders often can point a finger at substances in their blood to which they are sensitive and which trigger an immune response. Blood is a huge reservoir of impurities, and although the body is designed to help filter, neutralize, and eliminate these impurities, today we tend to overload the body with too many to process on an ongoing basis. And once this ama—this bank of biomolecular sludge that antagonizes healthy biochemistry and our physiological systems—starts to build and block natural pathways, the ultimate insult sets in regardless of your unique dosha: inflammation.

The Destructive Fire in Inflammation

One of the most breakthrough discoveries in Western science during my career has been the revelation that the cornerstone of most diseases and degenerative conditions, including being overweight or obese, is inflammation. And by now the general public has a rough idea about "inflammation" in terms of the body. Whether it's the redness that quickly appears after a paper cut or the chronic soreness of an arthritic joint, it's commonly understood that when the body experiences an insult or injury, its natural response is to create swelling and pain, hallmarks of the inflammatory process. But inflammation isn't necessarily "bad." It's a signal that the body is defending itself against potential harm; it's a natural part of the healing process. When it's tending to an open wound or cluster of cancer cells forming a tumor, it's ultimately helping us to survive.

The problem with inflammation, which gives it such as negative reputation today, is that it can get out of control. A fire hose turned on momentarily to douse nearby flames is one thing; but leave the hose on indefinitely, and you've got another problem on your hands soon enough. And that's the case with inflammation gone awry. It's intended to be a spot treatment, not an ongoing process left on forever. But millions of people are besieged by an inflammatory process always in the "On" mode today. I see it every day in my patients. And it's rarely confined to one particular area, as the bloodstream allows it to spread to every part of the body; hence, we have the ability to detect this kind of widespread inflammation through blood tests to look for molecules indicative of the inflammatory process. Many of the biological substances produced as a result of inflammation run amok are toxic to cells, leading to cellular dysfunction and destruction. It's no wonder that people with high levels of inflammation have an extensive list of symptoms: fatigue, low resistance to infection, muscle weakness, joint pain, digestive disorders, acne, anxiety, headaches, depression, allergies . . . and body-weight chaos. They are also at a much higher risk for many illnesses, from diabetes and cancer to heart disease and dementia.

Today the leading scientific research shows that inflammation is a fundamental cause of the morbidity and mortality associated with all manner of disease and virtually every chronic condition you can imagine. In fact, we're beginning to understand that coronary artery disease, a leading cause of heart attacks, may actually have more to do with inflammation than it does with high cholesterol.

And obesity could very well be the outcome of chronic inflammation, not just ingesting too many doughnuts and sodas (though these foods trigger inflammatory pathways, hence their connection). In fact, new guidelines emerged in 2013 regarding the use of statins for people at risk of developing heart disease and stroke. Statins are prescription drugs used to lower people's cholesterol, but they are also incredibly powerful inflammation reducers and likely reduce the risk of not just cardiovascular disease but *any* disease. Developed by the American College of Cardiology and the American Heart Association, in collaboration with the National Heart, Lung, and Blood Institute, these new guidelines highlight the power of controlling inflammation for increased longevity. (The move was controversial to be sure, for it means millions more Americans should be taking such a drug in addition to paying attention to their diet and exercise habits. The decision to add a statin to your regimen is one that should be discussed with your doctor in light of your personal risk factors; statins are not side-effect free. You can do a lot to reduce your body's inflammation through lifestyle practices alone, including the Hot Belly Diet's protocol.)

Although focusing on reducing inflammation might seem out of place in a discussion of weight loss, we know now that it underpins the very process of metabolic dysfunction and uncontrolled weight gain. The longer your inflammatory processes are turned on, the slower your metabolism, the weaker your ability to burn fat, and the longer it takes for you to even feel full. Historically, we ate food rich in ingredients that helped us to keep inflammation in check. But the food industry today manufactures a lot of these critical nutrients out of our diet, so we are left lacking the dietary weapons we need for optimal health and energy metabolism. And, as I've already stated, consuming processed nutrients in the form of a pill does little to stem the tide.

So what's the solution? A gentle rekindling of your agni, which is what the Hot Belly Diet does using specific ingredients that have been known to mankind for thousands of years and that satisfy all of your body's nutritional needs. Ayurveda acknowledges numerous ways to improve agni, which in turn aid in taming the bad kind of inflammation. Among these strategies are adding certain spices to foods, drinking hot teas infused with ginger and lemon, lightening the load you put on your digestive system with foods that are easily digested, and incorporating physical activity in your day to stimulate metabolic activity and increase the flow of agni throughout the body—all of which will be part of the Hot Belly Diet. You'll also learn how to establish many other habits that support a humming, balanced agni, such as maintaining a regular sleep schedule, spending time in nature, doing seasonal cleanses, and staying away from cold fluids. I'll discuss these in detail in Chapter 9.

You want a balanced agni that is neither too weak nor too excessive. Hence, we are improving the body's movement of nutrients and communication between cells and organ systems—we're reshaping and recharging the natural dynamics of the body. If you can support a humming, "hot" digestive fire, you can foster rapid weight loss and sparkling health. Simple as that. And, as we'll see in the next chapter, the quality of agni varies depending upon your dosha: vata, pitta, or kapha.

What's more, the Hot Belly Diet turns on the pathways in your body that help reduce inflammation. Interventions designed to lower inflammation using natural substances like those you'll find on this diet have been described in medical literature dating back more than two thousand years, but it is only in the past decade that we have begun to understand this intricate and eloquent biochemistry. And it's not just what you eat that can help you manage inflammation. You're going to learn about the latest studies demonstrating the ways exercise and sleep come into play, as these are important facets of maintaining the body's critical balance of ideal weight, health, and happiness. The moment I put someone on this diet, one of the first things I hear back is that it has more than a physiological impact. It has a tremendous psychological effect. And as you feel that physiological shift, you become mindful automatically and you start training your mind to ask yourself regularly, *How do I feel?* And that is the goal of an Ayurvedic approach. I want to put you in touch with your body in a uniquely special manner that allows you to gain ultimate control of your weight and well-being.

The Youth in Agni and the Age in Ama

Your aging process is directly correlated with your agni. As you get older, your fire naturally and inevitably becomes weaker. Yet this fire is what's keeping you alive, so how you maintain that fire is how you keep your quality of life. I see so many people who retire and suddenly have problems with weight and chronic conditions. What's happening is that their eating habits and patterns change and they don't respect the natural decline in their digestive fire. In the ancient tradition, it's said that once you reach your sixth decade, you should have two meals a day. After seventy, eat once a day, at brunch time.

It's also important to note that inflammation and ama share a vicious cycle. One feeds on the other, since once chronic inflammation sets in, ama can accumulate more easily as digestive and metabolic forces are compromised. Clearly, excess heat is not the cause of inflammation—it's the lack of a fully functioning digestive fire that fans the flames of inflammation. Anyone who thinks they have intolerances to certain foods can also blame ama as part of the problem.

The Fat in Flour and the Whole Grain Truth

It's common knowledge now, especially among chronic dieters, that white and processed flours are not so good for you and that whole grains are ideal. But what many don't realize is that even whole grains can be exceedingly deceptive. "Whole wheat/grain flour," for example, is typically processed and modified by the time it arrives in your kitchen (or mouth), perpetuating that sticky sludge. Gluten-free diets have become all the rage recently, and for good reason: Gluten is the sticky quality of protein in wheat itself, and is also found in related grains including barley and rye. It's similar to that of ama. If you have low-grade ama in your system, you can develop a resistance to gluten-containing foods whereby the body's immune system reacts negatively to any gluten consumed. Symptoms of a food allergy then surface. (The good news is that if you're sensitive to gluten or have been diagnosed with celiac disease, the Hot Belly Diet can work for you.) Keep in mind, too, that it's not just wheat that triggers digestive disorders; lots of other toxic habits are commonplace in people's eating.

Before someone experiences issues with gluten, however, a slow buildup of ama has occurred that eventually leads to an allergic reaction from the immune system. The digestive fire weakens to the point that the body cannot handle gluten. Or, consider a person who experiences gastrointestinal issues, such as gas and bloating, upon eating refried beans. Beans can be problematic for many people because they contain a rich combination of both starch and protein, plus lots of nitrogen. This isn't to say refried beans are bad, but when they are consumed by someone with a weak digestive fire, over time they can cause digestive challenges. You'd be surprised by what your body can handle (and what foods you can enjoy!) once you get your digestive fire up to speed.

All of this, by the way, is related to your state of mind. How well your digestive fire burns plays into how you feel. Just as the weather can make you happy or sad, so can the condition of your agni. The stronger your agni, the more you can manage mentally, physically, and in terms of digestion. But getting back to a robust agni requires that you lighten up your dietary intake and focus on foods in the right portions and at the right time of day that will rebuild your digestive fire while taking control of ama. Which is exactly what

Dead Foods, Dead Metabolism

Most Americans have never experienced true hunger. We are overfed and undernourished. When you start to make your digestive activity sluggish, you create these impurities—the ama—in your system. The body's energy doesn't move, and you start feeling tired, toxic, and slow. The fire stops burning. Like any roaring fire, you need air for the fire to burn, but most diets don't offer that rekindling. Many diets cater to taste buds and feeding you dead food—starving you to the core and dampening your fire further. It's like throwing a wet log onto a fire, which then smolders. No wonder caffeine and energy drinks are ever more popular. People are desperate to feel enlivened and light rather than dull and heavy. But such measures sustain a cycle of smog in the system rather than pure energy. An optimally functioning metabolism is a function of how strong your digestive fire is, as well as what you're putting into it to burn. The Hot Belly Diet teaches you how to reignite a dead metabolism and support the "ojas" of life.

the Hot Belly Diet is designed to achieve. The foods on this protocol are easy to digest and supply a wallop of nutrients to rekindle your agni while burning off that ama. In other words, we're resetting your body's ability to accept and assimilate the energy and nutrients found in food while giving it the tools it needs to burn the most calories and fat. And the whole grains recommended on this diet are the very ones that rigorous science has repeatedly documented to reduce your risk for many diseases while improving weight loss and maintenance.

Ojas: The Vital Energy of Life

To achieve optimal health, you must remove the ama pooled in your body and focus on producing *ojas*, a Sanskrit term meaning "vigor." Ojas is prime energy—the pure substance that's released from completely digested food. It moves throughout the body, helping to sustain its biology while bringing clarity to the mind and balance to the emotions. When your body creates ojas, you feel wonderful because your cells are singing with happiness. Ojas are a reflection of your mind and body getting the nourishment they need.

It follows, then, that to stimulate the generation and flow of ojas, you need a dietary protocol that concentrates on pure, "*sattvic*" foods, which the body can easily digest to release its ojas. The most sattvic foods include those found on this diet, notably seasonal fruits and vegetables, sprouted mung beans, and nuts and seeds. The foods that are difficult for the body to convert into ojas, including fatty meats, fried and processed foods, leftovers, canned or reheated foods, and excessively salty or sour foods, will be avoided. In addition, as you can imagine, certain lifestyle habits like smoking, consuming alcohol, and sitting all day also destroys ojas.

The chart on page 44 will help you gauge whether you possess healthy ojas or too much ama. If you've been storing ama, the Hot Belly Diet will begin to nourish you in ways that will tip the scales in favor of ojas and you'll soon enjoy increasing levels of joy and greater well-being.

What Lies Ahead?

I know you're wondering how fast you can lose the weight and what's realistic for you. Instead of thinking in terms of how many pounds you can drop, see if you can shift to the positive and ask: "What will I *gain*?"

Signs of Ojas	Signs of Ama
You feel rested upon awakening.	It's hard to get out of bed.
Your skin has a healthy glow.	You have tired, sallow skin.
You have clean breath and a pink tongue.	You have bad breath and a coated tongue.
Your body feels light, regardless of your weight.	Your body feels heavy.
You have a strong appetite.	You have a dull appetite.
You feel centered during your day.	You feel fatigued, spacey.
Your digestion is strong.	You have sensitive digestion, bloating, and sluggish elimination.
Your body feels robust and pain-free.	You have generalized pain.
You feel energized and optimistic.	You have difficulty realizing your intentions.
Your mind is clear.	You suffer from depression.
You rarely get sick.	You are susceptible to infections.

I won't sugarcoat the other truth that you should accept right now. I have no doubt that if you follow this diet to a T, you will lose weight. But you cannot find long-lasting success unless you factor in all the other elements of your lifestyle that can have a big impact in your weight-loss efforts. Your age, level of activity, job, day-to-day responsibilities, and overall stress contribute to the state of not only your physical body and fat-burning capacity (including the state of your agni and levels of ama), but also your state of mind and how you feel in that body. The agni can become weak or aggravated if you eat out of accordance with your constitution, or doshas, habitually eat the same foods, overeat, eat tasteless foods, drink too much water with meals, stay up late, eat at irregular times, resist the urge to eat, or don't exercise enough. Look at how many of these factors relate more with lifestyle than actual "diet" per se. The Hot Belly Diet affords you the opportunity to repair, rebuild, and maintain a thriving agni through various strategies that each target the health of your digestive fire from a different angle.

Following a specific dietary protocol is like spot-treating an ailment that should be addressed from a broader perspective. Although most diets (especially those that are marketed to detoxify your body) promise "total body rejuvenation," rarely do they entail a program that can achieve such a monumental change. In ancient Indian philosophy, *kayakalpa* is a system of total body transformation that takes about three months of focus to rebuild one's entire body; at the heart of this transformation is the process of renovating one's digestive powers, which are seen as a center of gravity for all things health- and longevity-related. Today's *panchakarma* practices found in many spas and retreat centers reenact this old tradition on a shorter time frame. Panchakarma therapy is an ancient method of detoxifying the body through the use of oils, herbs, body treatment, meditation, and yoga.

One of the reasons I wrote this book is that I know that many people cannot take time away from their busy lives to move into a retreat center for a month (let alone three) and concentrate squarely on good nutrition, twice-daily yoga, and meditation. Which is why I've created this program to give you maximum results in the shortest period of time, while you go about your daily duties and do your best to make modifications to your lifestyle that aren't terribly difficult, but that can reap you enormous rewards. I will be asking you to start a yoga routine (all the details of which are in Chapter 7) and seriously consider the tips I've outlined in Chapter 9. Some of these strategies will be easy to implement, such as drinking warm water throughout the day and avoiding eating in front of passive entertainment like the TV or computer. But some, such as being strict with your sleep schedule and making lunch—not dinner—your most important meal of the day, will likely take time to get used to and master. And that's okay. I've included plenty of ideas for helping you to make these strategies doable and practical in today's world.

Unfortunately, we live in a mode whereby we expend our health to get wealth. By that I mean we tend to avoid taking care of ourselves the way we should as we chase success at whatever cost. Some of us think that "once I get to here" or "when I make X dollars," we'll be able to slow down and then begin to take better care of ourselves. But I don't see this happening. Good intentions of spending our wealth (once we have it) to regain health don't usually pan out the way we imagined. I see an untold number of people who reach their forties and fifties and are saddled with chronic illnesses or serious diseases that are not easily reversible, if at all. They may finally have all the money they need to take better care of themselves, but it's too late.

My goal for you is to avoid such a fate, as Mark did a few years ago. I first saw Mark when he was thirty-nine years old and living in the Midwest. He was working in a company doing global sales and dealing regularly with the Chinese market, and his job had him awake late in the night. He lived on snacks and junk food and, of course, lots of coffee. Once a month, he went to Sam's Club to load up on supplies. Although he wasn't severely overweight and didn't look that bad from the outside, his insides told a different story. He was prediabetic and had high cholesterol. One of the first complaints he had was a very low sex drive, which he thought played into his girlfriend's dumping him, something that further bruised his ego. He knew he needed to find a better job, so it was easy for me to suggest he quit. With my help, he cleaned up his diet and stopped snacking. He started consulting work and took to walking every day. Within a matter of months, he cultivated new habits that put him in prime health.

Months? But I thought this diet only took 30 days? It takes about a month to establish new habits, and the Hot Belly Diet can yield results in that time frame. But some of you may choose to continue the Accelerate protocol for longer than recommended (21 days) and reap greater benefits. Three cycles of the Accelerate Phase create a much stronger cellular memory in your body that can stand the test of time. At that point, when you begin to stray from newly formed habits, you notice it right away and actually begin to miss them. Which makes it that much harder to revert to old, unhealthy habits and erase all of your accomplishments.

In total, the Hot Belly Diet is a 30-day program—a core 21-day phase bookended by two short phases to gradually wean you from your current eating habits and then help you reach a maintenance phase in the final week. In general, if you're closer to your target weight, you will probably lose weight more slowly. This is to be expected. Don't be dismayed if your weight doesn't drop fast or significantly at first. Look for any progress, whether it be increased energy, losing inches around your waist (your clothes will start to loosen), or a brighter sense of self. But if you have more than thirty pounds to lose, chances are you will start seeing results rather quickly.

It's perfectly fine to focus squarely on the dietary protocol for the first month and then consider adding your exercise routine and the additional tips outlined in Chapter 9. Some people need to take intensive transformations one step at a time, and that's okay. For those who want to be ambitious from the start, adding a yoga and walking routine right away will no doubt accelerate your results. The beauty of this program is that you won't get discouraged or bored, and you can always come back to this 30-day protocol (or just the Accelerate Phase) whenever you feel like you need a reboot or you've gone too far off track. This can happen at various times in our lives, such as during the holidays, times of increased stress, or, conversely, during unique celebratory periods like weddings. You'll love the fact that in just a week you'll be slimmer and you'll feel a lot lighter and energetic. This will set the stage for even more dramatic changes ahead as virtually every cell—and cellular transaction—in your body undergoes a renovation. Among the immediate effects (some of which you may not necessarily "feel") that will be taking place over the next month are:

> Mobilization of fat stores so excess fat can be easily burned off.
> Higher-functioning digestion and metabolism so you can absorb nutrients better.
> Blood sugar balance.
> Removal of toxins that antagonize every system in your body, from digestive to immune.
> Lower levels of inflammation.

All of these positive effects translate to big payoffs that you will eventually feel, from physical sensations of optimal energy to a sense of peaceful well-being.

It is my belief that the concept of agni is one of the most overlooked and yet overpowering keys not just to balanced weight, but to health and longevity as well. I hope I've implanted a totally new idea in your mind that will allow you to once and for all take control of your health. Now let's get to the diet.

CHAPTER 3

Flow, Burn, and Build: The Goals of the Hot Belly Diet

To keep the body in good health is a duty . . . otherwise we
shall not be able to keep our mind strong and clear.

—BUDDHA

Last year, a forty-two-year-old man who ran a Silicon Valley IT company came to me for help in treating his chronic sinusitis. He was your typical type A personality, and I knew right away that he didn't want to be in my office and had reluctantly decided to see me based on a friend's urgent recommendation. This happens quite a lot—someone tries traditional medicine and then reaches out to me in a last-ditch effort. This man, whom I'll call Peter, had gained close to thirty pounds in the last five years, tipping the scales at nearly 230 pounds. His balloon-like face looked puffy, red, and flushed—all signs of his inflamed sinuses. He sat restlessly in the waiting room and didn't enjoy the task of filling out my standard consultation form that I have all new patients complete so I can gain information about their health history, objectives, general habits, and lifestyle patterns. In the section that addressed his diet, he listed restaurants instead of food. He left the questions about the times of day he typically ate and the queries about psychological stress totally blank. Once we were in the exam room together, he described how he'd wake up every morning feeling cloggy, dull, and congested. He'd "tried everything," including nasal decongestants, antihistamines, Claritin, nasal sprays, and a bronchodilator. He was also taking a painkiller for a joint condition that affected his back and knees. And when I asked about his energy levels, he admitted that they were low, as was his libido.

As with all of my patients, I first looked beyond his medical concerns and asked him questions that would give me a full picture of Peter's lifestyle. Peter was like so many other Silicon Valley work-aholics, with hundreds of people relying on him. In addition to eating at a lot of restaurants, he had a habit of putting little thought into the foods he was choosing at home. He woke up early in the morning each day to get a head start so he could beat the traffic. His breakfast consisted of coffee, eggs, bacon, toast, and OJ. He'd leave the house by 7:30 a.m., then sit most of the day in meetings. When I asked him about lunch, he said, "There's no real lunchtime. I'm busy all day. If I'm lucky, I grab a sandwich." In the evenings, he waited for the traffic to settle down before venturing home at around 8:00 p.m., after which he enjoyed a "banquet" of food prepared by his wife and downed a couple glasses of wine. Then, he scrolled through his email once more before another night of poor sleep. On weekends, he took his kids out for big breakfasts and typically found himself going out for dinner with his family on those nights, too.

Once I heard these details, I easily identified the problem. "Do you realize that you're eating the wrong foods at the wrong times of the day?" I asked him. But it wasn't what he wanted to hear, and neither was the solution. I then had to tell him that I didn't have a magic pill or elixir to give him, and that he'd have to change his schedule and diet to find relief. I used his dinner routine as an example, explaining: "You're sleeping with a big meal in your system. It doesn't get fully digested properly, which is why you wake with that heavy, congested, sticky feeling—which you then worsen with your heavy breakfast before sitting all day." I told him that he had to abandon the false idea that breakfast had to be "the most important meal of the day" and to try a small bowl of oatmeal in the morning, to eat a substantial organic lunch during the day that consisted of salad greens, vegetables, and a lean source of protein, and then come home to a simple bowl of brothy, hot soup.

"I didn't come to you for this!" he said angrily. Evidently, he wanted an exotic herb to cure him—not instructions (or criticism) on his diet. He refused to pay me and walked out.

You'd think that Peter would have vanished forever, but a funny thing happened. Just before he stormed out, I told him to come back in three weeks. He didn't make it that long. A mere two weeks later, he called my office insisting that I see him. He returned looking like a totally different person. Peter now had a twinkle in his eye. Despite his disdain for my "prescription" on that first day, he must have been desperate enough to try it. "My wife packed my lunch the first week," he said. "I ate soup when I got home. Within a few days, I woke up for the first time without feeling dull and congested. I actually looked forward to my bowl of oatmeal."

"Now we can finally talk," I said to him, describing the Hot Belly Diet that he was now willing to commence wholeheartedly. As it turned out, Peter's transformation was more than just his newfound desire for oatmeal in the morning and simple, easily digestible meals at lunch and dinner. His snoring halted, and his sex life and restful sleep returned. A month later, he'd shed close to twenty pounds. His face looked bright and clear, and he no longer needed to use his inhalers and medications. He went for walks in the morning before work, moved more throughout the day, and took an evening stroll. Everything in his life was better, and though it wasn't a surprise to me, he seemed to have a eureka moment when he commented, "I went to *so* many doctors, and nobody ever bothered to ask what or when I was *eating*."

Peter's story is emblematic of so many others' experiences. Here we have an intelligent, logical, successful person who ironically fails to understand some of the most basic facts of life: the implications of lifestyle choices. Despite the enormous array of health challenges that I see in my patients, the vast majority of them have problems that can be reduced to diet.

It's amazing to me that in the wake of this epidemic of obesity and chronic illness today, so few of us stop to think about how our diets factor into our well-being. It's human nature to prefer a short-cut and ask for a prescription or seek a potion that will wipe away our problems. Granted, there's work and effort involved in choosing to eat a certain way and avoiding the habits that get us into trouble to begin with, but when it comes to desperate measures, health challenges that disrupt our quality of life can provide enough motivation to change.

Making the decision to reorganize his lifestyle was perhaps Peter's biggest hurdle, for once he started my program, he found it easy to stick to it. He got a taste of health early on, and it infused him with more motivation to keep going. And that's key. The Hot Belly Diet will generate results in a reasonable period of time so you, too, can initiate a new pattern of healthy habits that lead to lifelong weight control. What follows is a careful look at the main elements that make the diet work.

The Ama Test

In the last chapter, I introduced you to the role that ama could be having on you right this minute. It's that slimy, sticky residue left behind in your body from poorly digested food. Sounds gross, and it is. If you're like most people I treat, the moment you hear about ama is the moment you immediately wonder how much you have in your body. Before you even begin the Hot Belly Diet, it helps to get a general idea of your current ama levels. There is no blood or other lab test that can give you a report. The best way to gauge your levels is to answer a few basic questions, which reflect the symptoms that emerge when the levels of ama increase beyond the body's ability to deal with it.

For each question below, rate your matching characteristics on a scale of 0 to 5: 0–1 for "doesn't apply"; 2–3 for "sometimes applies"; 4–5 for "strongly applies."

1. My body feels clogged sometimes (e.g., constipation or congestion).
2. I often feel gassy and bloated or get heartburn.
3. I sometimes wake with a headache.
4. I have low energy.
5. I often feel dull, heavy, lethargic, and unmotivated. (I don't have a passion for life like I used to.)
6. I often have to clear my throat because I feel mucousy.
7. It's hard for me to get through my day because I get tired.
8. I frequently feel dull and depressed. (I am unhappy.)
9. It's hard for me to taste food without adding salt.
10. I deal with health issues chronically.

Add up your total. A score between 1 and 19 indicates a low level of ama; between 20 and 34 indicates a moderate amount of ama; 35+ indicates a high amount of ama.

Another way you can easily diagnose ama is to simply look for it. Tomorrow morning, when you wake up, open your mouth in front of the mirror before doing anything else such as brushing your teeth, rinsing with mouthwash, or drinking water. If you notice a white coating on your tongue, that's it. That's ama, and if it's present on your tongue, then it's present throughout your physiology!

I want to emphasize that just as extra weight is always a sign of nutritional and metabolic imbalance, so is ama. And despite popular assumptions that say your weight (and I'll add ama here) is a factor of how much you eat and how much exercise you get, the truth is that these two barometers of health are influenced by *what* types of food you eat and in which *combinations, when* they are eaten, and how they are *digested and absorbed.* If any of these components are suboptimal, then the body will not be able to function well and your weight will suffer as ama accumulates. You could be eating organic healthy food, but in the wrong combinations at the wrong time of day—and your body knows it.

The Hot Belly Diet affords you the structure—and flexibility—you need to address all of these health components. Put simply, I'm going to show you how to fulfill the what, when, and how to stirring that fire in your belly, from which all paths to wellness and perfect weight commence. And by clearing the body of ama, you set the stage for vibrant health.

The Body's Clock: Keeping the Flow

The Hot Belly Diet honors the body's internal clock. In Ayurveda, there are certain times of the day when it's ideal to consume foods, and other times that should never entail eating. In fact, harmonizing our internal rhythms with those of nature improves daily self-renewal on both a cellular and emotional level. This isn't based on some anecdotal idea passed down through generations; we know now that we're programmed to physiologically respond to a day/night cycle based on the twenty-four-hour rotation of the planet. Our bodies have evolved to respond to the solar day's cues by eating and pursuing activities during daylight and to rest and sleep during darkness. The science of chronobiology has actually managed to identify the exact genes that control this circadian clock, and one in particular that commands our body's sleep-wake rhythms throughout the twenty-four-hour day is aptly named the clock gene. (In addition to our circadian rhythm, there are other recurring cycles in nature that Ayurveda respects, such as the seasonal rhythm, the twelve-month cycle of the earth around the sun; the lunar rhythm, the monthly cycle of the moon around the earth; and the tidal rhythm, or the gravitational influence of the moon on water.)

The urge to sleep after the sun goes down and to be active during the day is a prime example of your inner ticktock. But there's much more to this biological timekeeper than just helping us keep track of when we should be alert and when we should welcome periods of rest. It has built-in mechanisms to control a wide array of functions, including those that help us to stay lean and fit. It impacts our metabolism, moods, and immune system. We're just beginning to understand the many ways it commands our health. In 2012, for example, researchers in Georgia found that a part of this master clock gene, which helps regulate the cardiovascular system, does not function properly in obese animals, as it does in non-obese animals. This helps explain why obese individuals usually have disrupted circadian rhythms, triggering them to eat at irregular times, and especially late at night. Not only does this lead to a bad night's sleep, but often these people also suffer from sleep apnea, a condition that further interrupts their sleep rhythm. Shift workers who start their day at 9:00 or 10:00 p.m. at night tend to be obese because their physiological requirements are backward. And those who alternate their night shifts on a weekly basis, switching to a day shift for a week, are known to be at a much higher risk for obesity. These individuals' physiological cues swing back and forth, interfering with their natural circadian rhythms. All of this, unfortunately, keeps unrestrained inflammatory pathways on, leading to those feelings of heaviness and lethargy, and congestion in the morning.

So while it's true that calories cannot tell time, the body indeed can tell time. Calories are received by the body differently depending on a variety of factors, including—you guessed it—the time of day. Even though Peter deprived himself at work by not eating much and then came home to a bounty of calories his body needed, he was doing a disservice to his agni by catering to it at the wrong time and with an overabundance of foods difficult to digest. His habits were, in effect, killing his digestive fire and contributing to a buildup of intestinal sludge that was feeding his chronic sinusitis.

No sooner did Peter begin the Hot Belly Diet than he watched all of his symptoms disappear. And the one strategy that I made sure he prioritized above all others on the program was to put lunch on his agenda every single day no matter what. I even went so far as to recommend that he set the alarm on his watch and have his midday meal already prepared.

Lunch—not breakfast—should be the most important meal of the day. In fact, the importance of eating lunch before 3:00 p.m. was just recently proven by the first large-scale, long-term study ever performed to verify the common belief that it's better to have your biggest meal earlier in the day. The researchers, a combination of scientists from Spain's University of Murcia, Boston's Brigham and Women's Hospital, and Tufts University, just outside of Boston, conducted their study in the Spanish seaside town of Murcia. Lunch happens to be the main meal of the day in Spain. And what they found, surprisingly, is that all things being equal (including the number of total calories eaten daily, sleep quantity, and activity levels), the people who ate lunch later in the day had a harder time losing weight. All of the participants in the study were either over-weight or obese, and they were put on the same five-month weight-loss program. Half of the 420 participants that usually ate lunch after 3:00 p.m. lost an average of seventeen pounds. The early din-ers, on the other hand, lost an average of twenty-two pounds on the same diet. These results were published in the *International Journal of Obesity* in January of 2013.

Although we intuitively know that it's best to avoid bingeing on calories toward the end of the day, when we're tired and less ac-tive (not to mention our metabolism is slowing down as part of the body's natural circadian rhythm), so many of us fall into patterns whereby we prioritize lunch last. Our modern lifestyle is to blame; we're usually busy during the day and at the mercy of work schedules that don't let us plan lunch. So we end up either skipping it entirely or grazing on nutrient-poor snacks and food products until we can arrive home, slow down, and feast at the dinner table with multiple portions, dessert, and alcohol. (And for those who eat a big breakfast, skimp on lunch, and gorge at dinner to make up for those lost calories during the day, I can't even begin to describe what you're doing to your health.)

The Hot Belly Diet avoids this vicious, fire-quenching cycle by encouraging a wholesome lunch that has many benefits and is easy to prepare whether you're at home or on-the-go. As noted earlier, it's called khichadi, and it takes center stage during the Accelerate Phase of the diet. A delicious Indian comfort food that's been prepared for thousands of years, khichadi may well be the finest therapeutic recipe of all because it nourishes the entire system while enhancing the body's digestive fire. In fact, khichadi is so pure and nutritious that it's the first solid food that babies are introduced to in my native country of India. Its healing properties make it the meal of choice for the sick. And for the everyday person just looking for a burst of health in a bowl, khichadi fulfills that need.

What exactly is khichadi? You'll get the step-by-step cooking instructions in Chapter 4, but in brief, it entails a unique blend of protein, fat, carbohydrates, fiber, raw oil, vitamins, and minerals that feed the intestinal fire and supply all of the body's nutritional needs. You probably already have many of the ingredients to make this dish in your kitchen. My guess is you'll be surprised at how easy it is to prepare and take with you to work in a thermos to be consumed later in the day (which is what Peter did). On the Hot Belly Diet, you'll have up to two bowls of this superfood a day—a hearty one at lunch and a lighter version of it at dinner—each of which can be prepared in a slightly different way to offer variation. You can swap a bowl of khichadi with other meal options for those who choose to do so.

Don't panic at the thought of eating the same thing every day on this diet. You won't be, because you'll rotate your base ingredients (i.e., mung beans, basmati rice, buckwheat, and quinoa), as well as seeds (i.e., sesame, chia, and pumpkin), leafy greens (i.e., spinach, broccoli, kale, Brussels sprouts, chard, and cauliflower), and spices. I'll also allow you to incorporate lean sources of protein and fresh fruit. You, and your taste buds, won't get bored on this diet. These ingredients equip you with the perfect formula for keeping your digestive fire burning bright and using calories efficiently. Your emotional well-being will get a boost as well.

Not many people understand how food profoundly influences our mental state and emotions. That said, some are increasingly aware of the connection between eating too much sugar and feeling hyper, or the heavy, dull feeling from consuming too much dairy, fat, and red meat. By the same token, eating too many raw foods, and relying on juicing or a vegan diet rich in vegetables alone can leave one feeling spacey and unable to focus. Volumes have been written about an entire disease complex popularly known as "Syndrome X" or "Metabolic Syndrome," which is a group of risk factors involving erratic blood sugar fluctuations (an early sign of diabetes), high blood pressure, excess belly fat, high levels of blood fats, and low levels of good cholesterol. Khichadi positively addresses all of these physical conditions by optimizing blood chemistry. Which is partly why a greater sense of inner calm and peaceful well-being is one of the first notable experiences on this diet. You may even feel this within three days after beginning the protocol. You'll notice that your overall mood is better, that you don't feel like you're on the edge of a meltdown because of all the "to-dos" on your plate, and that you can succeed on this plan for the long haul. Put simply, the optimistic feelings will motivate you to keep going; your efforts will, in a sense, feel effortless!

The Health in Hunger: Creating a Burn

Several times a week, I correct someone for saying a version of the following: "But I thought it was important to stay semi-full throughout the day and graze on multiple meals rather than three large ones. Doesn't this keep the metabolism humming? Isn't it healthy to spread out my calories throughout the day and eat constantly?"

Quite the contrary: The more meals you eat, no matter how small (snacks included), the smaller your digestive fire will be.

Of all the lessons in this book, one of the most important takeaways goes against conventional dieting wisdom that says you should "never wait until you're hungry to eat." This is perhaps one of the most harmful pieces of advice out there in diet circles. Hunger is a vital marker of health. Appetite is your friend, not your enemy. It's imperative to experience a healthy sense of hunger between meals; one needs to prepare the body to receive food.

As I briefly noted in the first chapter, in Ayurvedic medicine, the secrets to speeding up your metabolism encompass deepana, which means "bioactivator," and pachana, which means "bioaccelerator." As these words suggest, the goal is to activate and accelerate your body's processes so that everything runs smoothly and efficiently. And this starts simply with digestion where you stimulate appetite and prepare digestion to extract nutrients quickly and easily once food arrives. This partly explains why calories are less of an issue if your digestive fire is strong—the calories you consume can be processed efficiently. People who graze all day and never get truly hungry are sapping their digestive fire. Think about it: If you're slowly putting fuel inside your body when you don't need it, excess fuel will get stored (as fat) and ama will begin to build. The fire begins to act more like smoldering embers rather than a hot flame.

If you've gone on diets before, then at one point you were probably told to eat five or six small healthy meals during the day to keep your metabolism in gear. You were persuaded to believe that eating routinely supported calorie-burning, and that any sensation of hunger triggered alarms in the body that translated to storing fat and slowing down metabolism.

We've come a long way in the advancement of mankind, but from an evolutionary standpoint, our DNA isn't too different from what it was for our ancestral hunter-gatherers. Contrary to what you may have been told, our ancestors didn't eat six times a day. For them, long periods of time without food were common. In fact our survival as a species is largely due to our ability to endure famine. Many cultures around the world still practice two to three meals a day without snacking. Many also encourage intermittent fasting, a long-established way of physically rebooting the metabolism, promoting weight loss, and even increasing mental clarity and insight (and this latter fact makes sense from an evolutionary standpoint: When food was scarce, we needed to think fast and smartly to find our next meal!). Although religions have maintained for centuries that fasting is good for the soul, the scientific evidence has been accumulating in just the last hundred years or so. In the early 1900s doctors began prescribing it to treat disorders like epilepsy, diabetes, and obesity. But today we have an impressive body of research to show that intermittent fasting, which includes everything from periodic fasts lasting a few days to merely skipping a meal or two on some days of the week, can increase longevity and delay the onset of diseases that tend to cut life short, including dementia and cancer. The exact mechanism is still an active area of research, but we think that part of the benefits stem from the creation of certain biomolecules during the fast that ultimately protect the body. Intermittent fasting mildly stresses the body, resulting in a revving of your body's cellular defenses against molecular damage or cell death. We know, for instance, that fasting triggers higher levels of brain-derived neurotrophic factor (BDNF), a protein that helps prevent brain cells from dying. Low levels of BDNF are associated with numerous brain-related disorders, from depression to Alzheimer's disease. Fasting also ramps up your body's ability to remove damaged cells and molecules. Moreover, it's famous for increasing the body's responsiveness to insulin (hence its role in helping treat insulin resistance and diabetes). No joke: A recent study at the Salk Institute for Biological Studies in La Jolla, California, revealed that mice did not become obese or show dangerously high insulin levels after they fasted for the rest of each day following a fatty diet for eight hours.

Despite all this good news about intermittent fasting, in America we've created a culture of habitual eaters and snackers 24/7. We've simultaneously created a culture of chronic conditions, including obesity. My heart sinks when I see frequent eating touted as a health-beneficial practice. Now that food is accessible virtually everywhere, we can hardly tolerate missing a meal. And we've deceived ourselves into thinking that hunger is the enemy and that grazing is good. This couldn't be further from the truth.

Experts recommending six meals a day claim that eating roughly every three hours will improve your metabolism, control blood sugar, decrease cravings, and spur weight loss. But scientific studies don't support these claims. In fact, medical literature has proven otherwise. In 1997 the *British Journal of Medicine and Medical Research* conducted a thorough review of all studies that examined whether or not frequent eating fueled the body's metabolism and spurred weight loss; it didn't find any evidence that eating six meals a day boosts metabolism, fat burning, or weight loss. According to the American Dietetic Association (ADA), if you eat more frequently when you're just slightly hungry, your risk for overeating is higher. It's clear that we can forget about that strategy. And what about the idea that frequent meals help control blood sugar? Indeed, eating mini meals throughout the day may make you feel more stable in the short term, but in the long term, this will backfire. When you eat every two to three hours, your body becomes dependent on a continual supply of food. So you'll lose an innate ability to endure missing a meal, and, as a result, your blood sugar will crash.

The New York Academy of Sciences published a report in 2002 stating that grazing all day long can put one at risk for type 2 diabetes, heart disease, and stroke. Why didn't you read that study? Because the lobbying from food manufacturers that say grazing is good (especially on their beautifully packaged products and tantalizing snacks) is a powerful one. We're taught to think that grazing is healthful dietary medicine, and we forget that people with blood sugar issues are typically eating meals full of refined carbs, sugars, stimulants, and unhealthy fats.

Here's another way to understand this cause-and-effect. When the body is fed every two to three hours, it uses fuel from those meals rather than burning its fat stores. So the body adapts to being spoon-fed consistently without needing to dig into its fat storage. Conversely, when you eat three meals a day and don't snack in between, the body is forced to turn to fat. When your body uses fat as an active fuel, you will experience increased energy, ability to focus, stable moods, better sleep, fewer cravings, and, of course, effortless weight loss.

The idea that less—eating fewer meals as opposed to many mini-meals even if the total calories adds up to be the same—really is more when it comes to weight loss was further put to the test when a study came out in 2013 proving the power of just two meals a day. As reported by NBC News, the study was presented at the American Diabetes Association conference, revealing that people with type 2 diabetes who consumed two large meals a day lost more weight than when they ate six smaller meals *with the same total amount of calories*.

The researchers, led by Hana Kahleova of the Institute for Clinical and Experimental Medicine in Prague, told the fifty-four study participants to choose one of two types of eating plans for twelve weeks: either six mini-meals or just large breakfasts and lunches. Both diet regimens reduced each person's intake by five hundred calories but they entailed the same nutrient and caloric content. Registered dietitians regularly met with the volunteers and half of them were given all of the meals. Although the people lost weight under both eating plans, those eating a big breakfast and lunch experienced more weight loss than those eating the six smaller meals.

In reality, it's too hard for most of us to cut out dinner entirely and rely just on two meals a day. The practical takeaway here is not so much about skipping dinner as it is eating more during midday and less frequently overall, which is exactly what the Hot Belly Diet is going to train your body to do without feeling deprived. Previous studies have already shown that if you ate three times a day, you'd receive the same benefits of eating just two times. So it's really minimizing how often you eat, because you'll tend to eat less overall. The Hot Belly Diet encourages a nutritious breakfast, a hearty lunch, and a lighter dinner with no snacking in between.

The Burning Hours

The period between dinner and breakfast is a critical time to burn fat, lose weight, refresh the body at a cellular level, and reboot a stable nervous system to handle the stress of the next day. This is why the Hot Belly Diet encourages a light meal for dinner that's easily digested so you're ready for sound sleep by 10:00 p.m. As we'll see in a later chapter, the body is most efficient at detoxifying and rejuvenating cells between the hours of 10:00 p.m. and 2:00 a.m., which is why it's critical to be asleep during those hours. This is also the time period during which the immune system can refresh itself.

If you're accustomed to eating multiple meals a day, the Hot Belly Diet will be a transition. But I trust you can do this given the satiety factor you'll experience at each meal. Once your body gets used to this new routine, you'll never think about snacking again. You'll come to appreciate, enjoy, and happily anticipate that sense of hunger in between meals. Try not to stray from my guidelines and recommendations. After all, the goal of the Hot Belly Diet is to return your body to its more natural state where you can burn fat easily and steadily. For those who want to accelerate the entire process from the get-go, I'll explain how you can use a castor oil cleanse prior to beginning the diet. This can help jump-start the body's ama flush and promote quicker results.

The Carb Conflict

Another popular diet myth says that restricting carbohydrates can not only help you lose weight, but also improve your general health. In truth, your weight is a result of how many calories you consume versus burn on a daily basis. If you cut carbs, especially over the long term, you could rob yourself of significant nutritional benefits.

When people ask me for my secret formula for weight loss, I am met with disbelief when they realize it's based on carbs. How can the body burn fat when you eat carbs? In recent times, we've come to demonize carbohydrates and regard them as a source of calories that quickly convert to fat. How can I explain this conflict?

It's a shame carbohydrates have been relabeled as fattening. Anyone who has gone on a low-carb diet knows how difficult it can be. There's only so much protein and fat one can eat before the innate craving for carbs kicks in. And this instinctive craving is indeed part of our makeup, for carbs are a pivotal source of nutrition for a variety of reasons. Let me list the top seven:

Reason 1: Carbohydrates are your body's chief source of energy. No less authority than the Mayo Clinic asserts this. Carbs are comprised of sugars that break down to provide energy. So-called simple carbs, such as those found in most fruits and vegetables, are sources of quick energy. Complex carbs, on the other hand, like those in fiber-rich whole grains, supply longer-lasting energy. In addition to delivering the energy the body needs to run, carbohydrates also feed and fuel the brain. The brain prefers glucose because it's the only substance its cells normally use (brain cells cannot directly use fat for fuel).

Reason 2: Carbs will boost your mood and preserve memory. Although anecdotal evidence tells you that restricting carbs will leave you cranky, tired, and fuzzy-minded, it's a proven fact. Researchers suspect that carbs promote the production of serotonin, a brain chemical tied to feel-good emotions. In a 2009 study published in the *Archives of Internal Medicine,* people who went on a very low carbohydrate diet for a year experienced more depression, anxiety, and anger than those who followed a low-fat, high-carb diet that revolved around whole grains, fruit, legumes, and low-fat dairy.

In a 2008 study from Tufts University, overweight women who followed a no-carbohydrate diet for a week performed worse on memory tests than their counterparts who followed a low-calorie diet based on American Dietetic Association guidelines. If carbs make you feel dull, lethargic, and mentally foggy, then I challenge you to try my diet first and see if you still experience those symptoms. Chances are, the carbs that gave you trouble in the past didn't resemble those found on the Hot Belly Diet. Not all carbs are equal. (For those who truly think they are "carb-sensitive" and are concerned about this diet, see the box on page 68.)

Reason 3: Carbs can promote weight loss and prevent weight gain. In 2009 researchers at Brigham Young University in Utah published their results in *The Journal of Nutrition* after they followed the eating habits of middle-aged women for nearly two years. They found that women who boosted their fiber intake by eight grams for every one thousand calories consumed lost about four-and-a-half pounds over the course of the study (this was true whether they were eating five or twenty-five grams of fiber per day at the start of the study). It's virtually impossible to consume natural fiber from protein and fat. Instead, we get our fiber from other sources of carbohydrates—mainly vegetables, fruits, and grains. Studies show that when you meet fiber recommendations (healthy women should aim to get twenty-two to twenty-eight grams of fiber daily, and men should try to get twenty-eight to thirty-four grams), you can improve digestive health as well as lower your blood cholesterol and blood sugar levels. What's more, carb-rich whole grains, fruits, and vegetables can fill you up on few calories and keep you satisfied for extended lengths of time. Which is why these foods aid weight control.

The khichadi dish provides fiber from natural sources to keep your digestive system running fast and smoothly. You'll get your fiber requirements on this diet without having to count grams or even think about it.

Reason 4: Carbs help regulate your body weight, shrink belly fat, and protect your heart. Several studies have emerged recently to show that swapping refined grains for whole grains may help reduce total body fat and belly fat while protecting the heart. Just this year, *The Journal of Nutrition* published findings by Danish researchers that demonstrated how postmenopausal women who exchanged their refined grains for whole grains over the course of twelve weeks experienced a significant drop in body fat (3%). Those who continued to eat refined grains didn't lose as much fat. What's more, the whole grain group also experienced a notable drop in cholesterol, which wasn't seen in the refined grain group. The protective effect that whole grains can have on the heart has been established by other studies, and now research indicates that upping your soluble-fiber intake (a type of fiber found in foods like oatmeal and legumes) by five to ten grams each day could result in a 5 percent drop in "bad" LDL cholesterol. Similarly, people who eat more whole grains (e.g., brown and wild rice, buckwheat, quinoa) also tend to have lower LDL cholesterol and higher "good" HDL cholesterol. The Hot Belly

Confusing Carby Vocabulary

It's common to see terms such as *low carb* and *net carbs* on products, especially those affiliated with a certain diet program. The Food and Drug Administration, however, doesn't regulate these terms. *Net carbs* refers to the amount of carbohydrates in a product minus fiber or both fiber and sugar alcohols.

According to the Mayo Clinic, the glycemic index (GI), another popular term, classifies foods according to their potential to raise blood sugar. Many nutritious foods, such as whole grains, legumes, vegetables, low-sugar fruits, and certain dairy products, are low on the glycemic index. Weight-loss diets based on the glycemic index typically limit foods with a relatively high GI ranking, such a brown rice, potatoes, and raisins. But there are health benefits from many of these foods, so you don't necessarily have to eliminate them entirely from your diet. The GI can be an inaccurate tool to use in regulating your diet, because the entire chemistry of a meal can change depending on how you're mixing and matching various ingredients. You can turn a high-GI meal into a low-GI meal just by adding more fiber and healthy fat and protein. So we won't be using references to the GI while on the Hot Belly Diet. You needn't even think about it regardless of what other diets have taught you.

Diet features whole grains in combination with the right sources of protein and healthy fats.

Reason 5: Carbs will help you burn fat. Eating complex, "slow-release" carbohydrates, which is what the Hot Belly Diet features, fosters the burning of more fat, especially when you combine those slow-release carbs with the right proportions of protein and helps them gain better control of their condition and in some cases eliminate it.

I'll be offering you plenty of guidance throughout the program to address any personal issues that might arise while following the plan. I'll share a set of strategies to consider in tailoring the program to your body's needs as you slowly make the shift to a new way of eating. This will include the use of two natural supplements you've probably never heard about before. As Chapter 4 describes in detail, *triphala* and *trikatu* are ancient digestive gems that are finally available in the West and will help anyone to optimize their metabolism and weight-loss goals. I recommend that you take 500 mg of each twice daily during the diet and consider making these supplements a regular part of your routine even once your weight goals have been reached. Anyone who scored high on the ama test should most definitely consider these supplements, which target a sluggish digestion and the buildup of ama.

Bear in mind that we are changing your body all the way down to its cellular and biochemical makeup. It's a step-by-step process. All I ask is that you stay the course! Within a matter of days, you will start to notice a positive difference.

healthy fats and then exercise within three hours afterward. We've known for a long time that eating slow-release carbohydrates like whole grains and leafy vegetables doesn't cause a spike in blood sugar as high as eating refined carbohydrates, such as white bread, rice, and pasta. As a result, insulin levels remain well-managed— they won't signal your body to store fat, which in turn helps you to burn fat.

Reason 6: Carbs help prevent disease. Many carbohydrate-rich foods have the potential to reduce risks for chronic conditions and illnesses, including constipation, diverticulitis, birth defects, and heart disease. How so? Because these foods naturally contain vitamins, minerals, and nutrients such as B vitamins, iron, selenium, and magnesium, all of which contribute to cutting the risks of these conditions. These ingredients can be hard to come by in other foods and are easily assimilated into the body from natural carbs rather than synthetic supplements.

For those who worry that any grain, whole or processed, can be bad for health following reports that all carbs are bad, let me be clear: When the American Society for Nutrition invited researchers in 2010 to review the current scientific evidence regarding the health benefits associated with whole grains, they stated their findings quite bluntly for the prestigious *Journal of Nutrition* in a 2011 publication: Whole grains play a vital role in reducing the risk of chronic illnesses, from asthma to coronary heart disease, diabetes, stroke, and cancer; they are also instrumental in body weight management and gastrointestinal health.

Reason 7: Carbs help you feel satisfied. Let's face it: There's an innate satisfaction that comes with eating carbs. This is due to the feel-good hormones they release, as well as the warmth they can bring to your belly, both literally and figuratively. Most comfort foods are based on carbs, albeit the vast majority of the modern comfort foods are laden with too much sugar, white flour, processed fat, and salt that leave you overfed and undernourished. The khichadi dish is anything but. It's comprised of the highest-quality form of comfort—the kind that's rooted in the pleasures of nutrient-rich carbs that will promote your sense of fullness and speak healthfully to every cell in your body.

Of course, there's also something to be said for fats and proteins—both of which help you to burn stored fat when eaten in the right quantities, in the right combinations, and at the right time.

Determining Your Dominant Dosha

As I did with Peter and the individuals I introduced earlier, when I meet a new patient, one of the first things I do is determine the *essential nature* of that person. In other words, I don't concentrate on the details of their medical history and symptoms. That all comes later. First, I must decipher the most basic, yet critical, piece of information: What is the foundation of this person's mind-body system? The answer to that question is the only way I can help them get in touch with their inner intelligence, which is the true source of everything that comprises—and dictates—their life.

Consider, for a moment, some basic differences between you and a friend. Perhaps you're the type who drinks coffee and barely feels its effects, whereas your friend gets jittery and can't sleep well that night. You're the type who is easily chilled by a dip in the weather, while your friend doesn't notice. You like to keep a very rigid, well-planned schedule; your friend, however, flits throughout the day haphazardly and lacks organization. These variations cannot be identified by typical medical tests or body scans. They reflect certain characteristics and define our biochemical individuality. Ayurveda has organized this information into a system of psychophysiological body types. In fact, the word for body type in Sanskrit is prakriti, which literally means "essential nature." Your body type is your blueprint that outlines innate tendencies that have been built into every aspect of your mind-body system. Learning about your Ayurvedic body type will give you useful information on how to reawaken your body's inner intelligence and, more important, take advantage of that intelligence to lose weight.

We use the term *mind-body* a lot in my world. But the mind and the body are virtually one in the same. Every time there's an event in your mind, there's a corresponding event in your body. When you sense fear, for example, your body responds with adrenaline. Ayurveda looks at the meeting point between mind and body—the place where thought (e.g., fear) turns into matter (e.g., adrenaline in your bloodstream). And, according to Ayurveda, this interconnectedness is governed by three operating agents called the doshas. The doshas essentially facilitate the mind's dialogue with the body. Although I've mentioned the doshas in passing, let me define them at length here by giving examples of how they express themselves in real life.

If you're the type whose body is naturally slender and you like to be active, but can have irregular eating patterns and unpredictable sleeping patterns, I'd be able to identify which one of the three doshas was dominant in you: vata. Conversely, if you're someone who keeps a rigid schedule, complains when dinner is late, and enjoys intellectual stimulation, pitta is probably your dominant influence. And then there are those people who are somewhere in between—they are neither noticeably regular nor noticeably irregular in their personal habits and some describe them as easygoing. They tend to be more sedentary and don't like change. For them, a third dosha—kapha—is dominant.

My patients are often surprised by my ability to arrive at a deep understanding of their characteristics, both biological and psychological, based on a few questions about their eating and sleeping habits. For the record, Ayurveda isn't the only tradition that recognizes the existence of specific physiological categories. For centuries, cultures have created ways of describing different temperaments, different behavioral attributes, and even risk for disease. In medieval Europe, doctors described people in terms of their dominant "humor," which was derived from the natural elements of earth, air, fire, and water. Temperaments, behaviors, and even diseases were explained by an excess of one particular humor. Medieval medicine followed this tradition by aiming to balance the body's forces as dictated by the humors. In other words, a seventeenth-century doctor might have tried to make you less "melancholia" and more "phlegmatic." This approach has been replaced by modern medicine in much of the Western world. We didn't have to wait for today's technology, however, to tell us that heart attacks are more commonly seen in barrel-chested, hot-tempered males than in their trimmer, even-tempered counterparts.

Modern medicine may have its high-tech devices and sharper knives, but we all can appreciate different categories of people that reflect different types and corresponding risks to bear. Let's take a quick tour of the three doshas: vata, pitta, and kapha. Although they control thousands of separate functions in the mind-body system, they have three basic functions. Vata is like wind; it controls movement (its qualities are cold, dry, light, mobile, and erratic). Pitta is like fire; it controls metabolism (its qualities are hot, sharp, light, and oily). And kapha is like earth; it controls structure (its qualities are cool, moist, stable, heavy, and dense). Every cell in your body contains all three of these doshas. Just to stay alive, you need vata, or motion, to breathe, circulate blood, move food through the digestive tract, think and send nerve impulses to and from the brain. You need pitta, or metabolism, to process food, air, and water throughout your body. And you need kapha, or structure, to form muscle, fat, bone, and tendons and ligaments. Nature needs all three to build and maintain a human body. And, as I described above, just as there are three doshas, there are three basic types of human constitutions in the Ayurvedic system, depending on which of the doshas is dominant. Everyone is dominated by one, sometimes two, of these doshas. If I examine you and say, "You're a pitta type," I mean that pitta characteristics are the most prominent in you.

Below is a brief reference guide to the three doshas. Which one best describes you? This is not meant to be a scientific endeavor; you will likely find yourself exhibiting features from all types. More than anything, I want you to become aware of your most dominant dosha and tailor the program to your type. What's more, it's important for you to know which type of digestive fire you have (see the box on page 75) and how you will respond to this diet based on that knowledge.

(Note that the diet works *no matter what "body type" you have or which* dosha *is dominant*! I will make the individual tailoring of the diet to each body type easy and effortless with additional tips and strategies throughout the book.)

Characteristics of Vata Type

➤ Light, thin build
➤ Performs activities and walks quickly
➤ Irregular hunger
➤ Poor sleeper; tendency toward insomnia
➤ Enthusiasm, vivaciousness, imagination
➤ Excitability, changing moods
➤ Quick to learn new information, but forgetful
➤ Tendency to worry and overexert
➤ Tendency to be constipated
➤ Tires easily
➤ Mental and physical energy comes in bursts
➤ Imbalances associated with vata: accidents, Alzheimer's disease, arthritis, asthma, brittle bones, gas, pain

Characteristics of Pitta Type

➤ Medium build and strength
➤ Sharp hunger and thirst; strong digestion
➤ Tendency to become angry or irritable under stress
➤ Fair or ruddy skin, often freckled, with light or red hair
➤ Aversion to hot weather and sun
➤ Enterprising character, likes challenges
➤ Sharp intellect
➤ Precise, articulate speech
➤ Cannot skip meals
➤ Imbalances associated with pitta: heart conditions, skin rashes, blood and liver problems, acid indigestion

Characteristics of Kapha Type

➤ Solid, powerful build and strength
➤ Steady energy; slow and graceful in action
➤ Relaxed personality; not easily angered
➤ Cool, smooth, thick, pale, and often oily skin
➤ Slow to learn new information, but has a good memory
➤ Heavy sleeper; wakes up slowly
➤ Tendency toward obesity; seeks emotional comfort from eating
➤ Slow digestion, mild hunger
➤ Affectionate, tolerant, forgiving
➤ Tendency to be possessive, complacent
➤ Slow to make decisions; mulls things over
➤ Imbalances associated with kapha: obesity, depression, cancerous growths, asthma, diabetes

---

What Type of Digestive Fire Were You Born With?

Variable (vata): My hunger comes and goes; it's erratic and sometimes when I'm supposed to be hungry, I'm not. I can lose my appetite quickly.

Sharp (pitta): I can get ravenously hungry to the point I cannot wait for food.

Slow (kapha): I rarely feel ravenous. I'm more likely to feel low, dull, and sluggish after a meal.

Remember, I am not asking you to decode your dominant dosha like a scientist. Many people can identify with two doshas. I merely want you to be aware of which set of characteristics *most likely* reflects you so you can adapt the diet protocol maximally to your dosha. I'll be offering a few dosha-specific guidelines in upcoming chapters. The beauty of the Hot Belly Diet is that it's effective for every dosha and type of digestive fire. The bigger question you need to ask yourself at this point is whether you are ready. If yes, then take the following oath by repeating these statements:

> ➤ I will take my health seriously and modify my eating and health habits for life.
> ➤ I will prepare my meals at home and eat out less frequently.
> ➤ I will avoid "killers of digestion" during the diet. I will give up soft drinks, alcohol, processed flours, and refined and sugary sweets during the next 30 days.
> ➤ I will sip hot water throughout the day.
> ➤ I will accept the fact that this isn't just about looking or feeling better—it's about making a change in my life that will positively affect every aspect of who I am, from a spiritual, emotional, and physical standpoint.

I should add that our circadian rhythms follow doshic patterns as well. In other words, there are certain periods of time during the twenty-four-hour day that are governed by a particular dosha, and that can inform the ideal time to perform certain acts (eating, sleeping, exercising, working, meditating). I'll offer some advice in this regard in Chapter 9.

Holy and Unholy Waters

While following the Hot Belly Diet throughout the day, you'll get used to drinking hot liquids that stoke your digestive fire. Even after the diet, it's advisable to avoid cold or carbonated drinks, especially with meals. It takes five more minutes to digest any food you consume with a drink that's one degree below your body temperature (and for every degree below that, add five more minutes!). By sipping just hot water throughout the day, you help cleanse the digestive tract of blockages and impurities. Drinking hot water improves digestion and absorption of food, helping prevent the body from becoming clogged. It also mightily reduces cravings between meals. I have known people who lost over fifty pounds in a year by following only this single strategy!

Four of the main reasons why warm beverages trump cold ones is that, for one, they have a natural, mild vasodilatory effect (dilating the blood vessels and decreasing blood pressure), which has the upshot of increasing circulation to the gastrointestinal tract to in turn increase digestion efficiency while calming your nervous system. Secondly, hot liquids decrease mucous accumulation in your sinuses, throat, and gastrointestinal tract, thus decreasing the chances that invaders like viruses, bacteria, or fungi will grow or infect your body (hence part of the scientific reasoning behind chicken soup's profound healing properties). Thirdly, the temperature in our stomach is generally high, so it follows, then, that when we drink warm liquids during a meal, they help keep food in a semiliquid form, breaking it down more easily and helping to release it into the small intestine. And finally, warm water has been shown to increase body temperature and, as such, to slightly increase the metabolic rate. Although this minor metabolic boost might not be enough to actually cause weight loss, it likely can help the gastrointestinal tract and kidneys function better, a key to weight loss and overall health. I should also mention that warm liquids are just plain more enjoyable, at least to your brain. We have scientific proof now that when you drink hot water in particular, receptors in your mouth, throat, stomach, and intestines stimulate the pleasure center in the brain.

Most people can accomplish the hot water prescription by buying a good thermos and a small hot plate. You can pour your hot water into the thermos's cup, put it on the warmer, and sip it throughout the day as you work. Water that has been boiled for about ten minutes is the most purifying. The act of boiling water reduces its heaviness and energizes it. Avoid bottled water, including both spring and distilled; bottles pose a problem because they have been in transit during which heat could have leached chemicals from the plastic into the water.

The following fluids, which I call "unholy waters," should be strictly avoided for the duration of the diet:

➤ Coffee
➤ Carbonated drinks (including sodas, diet and regular)
➤ Energy drinks
➤ Alcohol
➤ Cold drinks of any kind (including fruit juice, flavored water, sports drinks, and sparkling water)
➤ Milk from cows, goats, and soy

The Hunger Meter

According to Ayurveda, a double handful of food is an ideal portion per meal (clearly, there are exceptions to this rule, especially when we consider leafy green vegetables that can be, by nature, voluminous; consider kale, spinach, or collard greens). I've already created this diet with built-in portion control given in the step-by-step instructions beginning in the next chapter. In general, however, the double-handful amount is a good measure to keep in mind; you'll use this amount to start and only go back for more if you're truly still hungry. How can you gauge this evasive feeling we call hunger? Use my "Hunger Meter" test, which outlines the spectrum of an eating experience.

First, place your hand on your belly to bring attention to that area. Then assess your level of hunger using the following:

Level 0: Your stomach is uncomfortably empty to the point you feel ravenous and don't care where your next meal comes from.

Level 1: Your stomach is empty and you sense hunger. You naturally gravitate toward food.

Level 2: You're eating and enjoying the food comfortably. You don't feel hunger, but you don't feel full either.

Level 3: You're starting to sense fullness coming on. You feel satisfied, but not stuffed. You know you could eat more, but you also know that you could stop and be okay. This is the level at which you should stop eating.

Level 4: You've gone beyond the level of comfort. You feel heavy, lethargic, and your belly is distended uncomfortably.

Level 5: You're stuffed to the gills. You cannot eat another bite and contemplate taking a nap!

It's important that you avoid levels 0, 4, and 5. See if you can stay between levels 1, 2, and 3. The goal is to leave your stomach partially empty at the end of your meal. This allows your digestive tract to work more effectively; your digestive furnace will stay aflame, and your body will find it much easier to control its weight naturally. Remember, being stuffed is not the same as being satisfied. In order to feel light, buoyant, energetic, and fresher the hour after you eat, you have to leave a little room in your stomach.

The Hunger Meter will be a tool you can use for the rest of your life. It's a simple method for checking in with your body and tuning into your true or false state of satiety.

Flow. Burn. Build. Those are the ultimate goals of the Hot Belly Diet. You're reinvigorating the natural, efficient flow of your body's energy, tapping its ability to burn fuel efficiently, and building healthy tissues through the flow-burn process. It's as simple as that. If it's been a while (maybe never) since you've gotten a diet to work for you, then let the Hot Belly Diet be your answer. And now that you're ready to get started, let's begin Phase 1.

CHAPTER 4

Phase 1: Prepare

DAYS 1–3

From food are born all creatures, which live upon food, and after death return to food. Food is the chief of all things. It is therefore said to be medicine for all diseases of the body and mind. Those who worship food as Brahman gain all material objects. From food are born all beings, which being born, grow by food. All beings feed upon food, and when they die, food feeds upon them.

—TAITTIRIYA UPANISHAD

It's long been known that food is medicine. Ayurvedic wisdom celebrates the "kitchen pharmacy," or the notion that simple food preparations, herbs, and spices can combat imbalances before they turn into full-blown illnesses. They also can, as you're about to find out, reboot the body in unimaginable ways, opening the door to not only a more disease-free life, but a mentally happier and physically thinner you.

As you begin the Hot Belly Diet, have a specific goal-weight in mind. And don't be unrealistic with the vision you have for yourself. You want to choose a goal that reflects a weight at which you feel vibrant and where you're happy with the way you look. For most people, this doesn't mean that the "perfect" weight rivals a supermodel's or allows you to buy a whole new size-zero wardrobe. I've treated as many patients who were underweight and felt terrible as much as I've encountered overweight individuals who feel fantastic. In truth, there really is no such thing as a perfect weight. We all come in different shapes and sizes, not to mention carry disparate sets of genes that code for various heights, body composition, bone structure, and even metabolism speeds. But there is a place of perfect health for every individual. That's what I want you to find—regardless of the number on the scale.

Although I don't normally give patients a specific goal-weight, as in "Let's get to 130 pounds," I do ask them to at least visualize what they will look and feel like once they reach their destination. Then they can come up with a rough target number on their own, one that they think will allow them to feel light, healthy, and energetic. If someone does have a specific goal-weight in mind when they come see me, I immediately ask: "Why is that number for you? What do you think you'll gain by being at that number?" My hope is that their response reflects worthwhile achievements such as alleviating or eradicating a chronic condition, having more energy to keep up with the family, or getting a good night's sleep every day.

Scientific studies show that seeing yourself in the shape you want to be in can help you reach your target. We all think in pictures, after all. So it helps to be able to keep a vivid image in your mind that serves to motivate and inspire you as you work toward achieving your ideal "picture of health." And again, try not to see yourself just gracing the cover of a magazine. Not that that's not feasible, but in reality, having a fit body is about being able to participate in life to its fullest and feel as fantastic as possible. So instead of a static cover model, see yourself engaged in the kinds of activities you want to do in a leaner, meaner frame that's beaming with boundless energy. Focus on what you'll gain in terms of energy, power, balance, and mental sharpness: You're active and playful with greater confidence and self-esteem. You're shopping at normal clothing stores and not thinking about people passing judgment on you. You're sleeping better, managing stress easily, and catching fewer colds. You're planning adventures and vacations that make physical demands of you. You're confident that you're doing the best you can to ward off illness and disease. If you deal with any chronic conditions, you're controlling them superbly and perhaps witnessing them have less of a negative impact on you. You're getting more done every day and feeling more accomplished both at work and at home. And you're enjoying life with your loved ones like you never have before. You may even want to write down your reasons for losing weight; rather than stating "I want thinner thighs and tighter abs," go for more ambitious, meaningful reasons like "I want to spend more quality time with my children," "I want to live longer," and "I want a better sex life." Think big picture.

How often should you weigh yourself? That's up to you, but I recommend that you don't get too caught up on stepping on the scale daily or even weekly at the beginning. It will take time for your body to ease into its new metabolic groove, and even though you'll likely be well on your way to shedding pounds from the first day as your body's internal chemistry shifts, you might not see that effect immediately on the scale. Remember, body fat is much lighter than muscle mass. As you burn fat and add more muscle mass, the scale can be deceiving. But you'll *feel* the difference in your clothing as well as in your mental clarity and level of energy. What's more, sometimes people's bodies retain more water when they begin to diet and as they train their bodies to accept a change in eating habits and their metabolisms undergo a rehab. Don't be alarmed if your weight goes slightly up on the scale early on during this diet; that uptick will reverse course as you continue, and then pick up speed. Also keep in mind that you're not just burning more calories and peeling away layers of excess fat around your waistline; you're positively affecting and modifying your metabolism, your motor skills and neurons, your organ systems—from digestion and skeletal to immune—your heart and lung capacity, your inflammatory pathways, and so much more. These cellular changes are much harder to track, but they are indeed happening deep inside.

That said, it's important to track your weight loss over the long term. Studies also reveal that tracking your weight is one of the most important tools you can use to manage weight loss and prevent weight gain (especially once you've lost it). I recommend that you weigh yourself and measure your waistline at the beginning of this diet for your start-up numbers and then at midpoint through the Accelerate Phase. Then you can weigh yourself again and measure your waistline at the end of Phase 2 prior to commencing Phase 3. If you find that your body isn't slimming down as fast as you'd like by the time you reach Phase 3, or you sense that you've hit a plateau somewhere, I'll give you some trouble-shooting ideas and guidelines that will help you move forward.

It helps to bear in mind that the human body is a dynamic, ever-changing machine. Just because you eat too many calories one day doesn't mean you'll wake up the next day ten pounds heavier. The body doesn't work like that. Everyone has days of minor derailments. I recommend keeping a daily journal to record what is happening in your life as you course through the program. This is where you can write down not only your reasons for weight loss, but your thoughts, track what life events are most affecting you—especially things that influence your dietary and lifestyle choices—and maintain an ongoing record of your emotions. Remember, your mental attitude has a lot to do with your body's weight maintenance. What's more, you can learn to use happiness as well as frustration as a motivator in your progress toward success. On those bad days that are inevitable, and that you wish to just forget about, aim to be extra vigilant about how those challenging moments affect those behavioral patterns that prevent you from being a healthy eater. Such self-awareness will help you to make positive changes.

My wish for you is that you learn a way of living that you can sustain for the long term. At this juncture, all I ask is that you make the most of these next 30 days and tune in to how your body is changing and feeling. You are recalibrating your body one day at a time and will see results relatively soon, and even more as those results accumulate over time. So take a deep breath, relax, and get ready to discover a whole new you.

Phase 1 Goals

The purpose of Phase 1 is to help you begin to extinguish old habits and wean your body from foods and drinks that dampen your digestive fire. It intends to lighten the load you put on your digestive system so it can heal and rejuvenate itself. You'll make incremental improvements in what you eat that build one day at a time in preparation for the Accelerate Phase. You'll also be given the opportunity to jump-start your weight loss with a twenty-four-hour cleanse that can accelerate your body's "reboot" and the rehabilitation of your digestive fire.

Phase 1 is titled "Prepare" for a reason: It primes your metabolism for rapid, but healthy, weight loss by igniting a new fire within your digestive system—your agni—while mobilizing that intestinal sludge, or ama, for permanent elimination. In doing so, it begins to detoxify your body to further support your digestive fire, correct improper digestion, and provide a solid foundation for a faster, more efficient metabolism. Phase 1 also removes the foods that trigger blood sugar imbalances and undeniable cravings. Once you evict the refined sugars and carbs that cause those ama-building surges in blood sugar, you can welcome the rewards that a healthy blood sugar balance brings to your biochemistry and mental clarity.

Phase 1 Protocol

Welcome to the training grounds. Now it's time to get started. I recommend that you plan to begin Phase 1 on a Monday or the first day of your workweek so you don't feel deprived. It's often easier to start a new diet while distracted by obligations at work than to try to commence a diet over the weekend amid social events. But if you're opting for the cleanse, then do that first over the weekend. Also use the weekend to prepare your kitchen—swapping out certain ingredients and buying replacements alongside your supplements (more on this below). You want to be ready to go come Monday morning.

Optional Twenty-Four-Hour Cleanse

Castor oil is a vegetable oil derived from the seeds of the castor-oil plant, which is indigenous to East Africa, but can be found growing in warm tropical regions throughout the world. Castor oil has long been known as a flushing agent for the gastrointestinal tract, as it cleans out and sanitizes the system—especially the gallbladder and liver, optimizing the flow of bile to boost digestion. For this reason, it's often recommended at the start of any health-improvement program and can further speed along results. It will also stimulate your body to burn fat and cleanse the deep tissues of your body. What makes castor oil unique is that it can affect the entire length of the bowel. It empties both the small and the large intestines. It also helps to prevent the absorption of liquids from the intestinal tract, which allows the bowel to retain more moisture and facilitate an easier passage of stool.

Since its first recorded use three thousand years ago during ancient Egyptian times, it's been a home remedy to relieve pain, increase lymphatic circulation, reduce inflammation, improve digestion, and treat everything from constipation to heartburn.

People under my care who follow the cleansing protocol rave about it one way or another. They love the way they feel—lighter and energized. The body will have eliminated a great deal of toxins and leftover sugars that have been clogging the system. It ultimately helps reignite a dead metabolism. The engines will start to run again.

Option: Fast for a Day

Want an alternative? Instead of the castor oil cleanse, you can choose to fast for a day and consume only liquids in the form of warm water, hot teas, and brothy soups. Fasting is an excellent, quick way to center yourself and get focused. As Plato once said, "I fast for greater physical and mental efficiency." And he wasn't joking. Fasting is a proven method to boost mental clarity and even metabolism. Contrary to conventional wisdom that says fasting lowers the metabolism and forces the body to hold on to fat in a so-called starvation mode, fasting provides the body with benefits that can accelerate and enhance weight loss, not to mention turn on DNA signals that ultimately lower inflammation. It is often said that fasting brings us closer to God and self-realization, while food indulgence drives us away. No wonder fasting has been an integral part of religious history. All major religions promote fasting as a spiritual practice: Muslims celebrate the fast of Ramadan and the Jewish community practices the fast of Yom Kippur. Yogis practice austerity with their diets, and shamans fast during their vision quests. In ancient Hinduism, the word *upavaas,* which is a one-day fast, literally means "to stay close to God." It also refers to staying close to yourself, to go inward. Fasting is also a common practice among devout Christians, and the Bible has examples of one-day, three-day, seven-day, and forty-day fasts. (I'll give some recommendations for intermittent fasting throughout the year in Chapter 9. Fasting can become an integral part of your ongoing health maintenance program.)

It is important to note that you can expect results in about five hours' time, but after the cleanse is over, you may not have another bowel movement the next day, since your system will have been cleared and must await the digestion of your next full meal.

If you choose to do this cleanse with the hopes of starting the diet protocol on a Monday, then make Saturday evening's dinner your last meal. (Tip: Avoid having a late and heavy dinner. And definitely do not engage in "last supper mentality," whereby you eat copious amounts of everything in sight and splurge on comfort foods fearing that you're about to be deprived.)

Then you'll get up early Sunday morning (between 6:00 a.m. and 7:00 a.m.) and drink the cleansing concoction. Here's the formula:

➤ Take two tablespoons (30 mL) of castor oil and mix it with half a cup of orange juice or grapefruit juice. Drink it all down. (Make sure the oil is fresh. For a list of recommended brands, go to www.hotbellydiet.com.) Some people do experience the urge to vomit, because as they drink it, they gag on it. But if you mix it properly, you should only taste the citrus.

➤ Consume only liquids for the remainder of the day. This can include liquid (meat-free, chunk-less) soups, stews, broths, freshly squeezed juices, and protein shakes. Avoid solid foods and vigorous exercise. Gentle exercises like walking and light stretching are fine. You will probably feel wiped out that day, and you will no doubt be spending time in your oval office (i.e., bathroom). Plan to stay at home or be within close range of a bathroom until your body is finished cleansing.

Some people don't respond to the oil cleanse within three to four hours, and in that case, just be patient. Sometimes it takes longer. (If nothing happens within two full days, then repeat the protocol.) But 80 percent of people will have loose bowel movements for several hours and be done by 2:00 p.m. Don't be alarmed if you experience explosive bowel movements; this is normal. A small percentage of people (5 percent) will have eight to ten bowel movements that day. Once the body quiets back down, you'll be poised to commence the Hot Belly Diet the following day.

Purchase Your Supplements

Every week it seems that we hear something in the media regarding the use of supplements. One day it's reported that certain vitamins are good for us and will extend our life; the next, we read about how some can increase our risk for certain diseases, including cancer, and cause more harm than good. While it's true that vitamins and supplements should never be used as an insurance policy against lapses in our diet, there's a time and place for some specific products that can help us in our weight-loss pursuits without any side effects or long-term risks. And there's a difference between mega-dosing on multivitamins and adding non-stimulatory natural supplements that the body won't otherwise obtain easily from the diet. There's also a difference between common Western supplements that rival many drugs and those endorsed by Ayurveda.

In addition to basic herbs and spices that humans have consumed for millennia, a number of Ayurvedic supplements comprised of plants and herbs have become widely available today. Two in particular have been a mainstay in Eastern cultures for centuries: *triphala* and *trikatu*. Thankfully, these digestive gems are finally available in the West and will help anyone to optimize their metabolism and weight-loss goals. Anyone who scored high on the ama test should most definitely consider these supplements, which target sluggish digestion and the buildup of ama.

TRIPHALA Triphala literally means "three fruits," because that's exactly what it is—an herbal formulation consisting of three fruits native to the Indian subcontinent: *amalaki, bibhitaki,* and *haritaki.* Triphala is most commonly known for its use as a rejuvenating tonic as well as a gentle, non-habit-forming laxative, which aids digestion, detoxification, and elimination. The combination of the three fruits helps many other systems as well, supporting the respiratory, cardiovascular, urinary, reproductive, and nervous systems. It can reduce serum cholesterol, improve circulation, reduces high blood pressure, and improve liver function. It's also been shown to be a powerful antioxidant, protecting cells from the damaging effects of free radicals.

Given all these benefits, it's no wonder that triphala is the most popular Ayurvedic herbal formula of India, and it's become one of the most valuable herbal preparations in the world. It's fast becoming a top herbal remedy in the western health food industry, especially given how many people suffer from chronic constipation and bowel irregularity. The three fruits involved in making triphala are also known for their individual effects:

➤ Amalaki (Emblica officinalis): This fruit, also known as the Indian gooseberry, has a cooling effect that manages pitta, supporting the natural functions of the liver and the immune system.

➤ Bibhitaki (Terminalia belerica): This fruit, also known as *Bahera,* is particularly good for kapha; it supports the respiratory system as well as kapha accumulations in the body.

➤ Haritaki (Terminalia chebula): Though having a heating nature, it is still good for all three doshas (vata, pitta, and kapha). It's known for its "scraping" effect, which helps remove toxins and helps weight maintenance.

In India we like to say: "No mother? Do not worry so long as you have triphala." In my culture, we believe that triphala is able to care for the internal organs of the body as a mother cares for her children. Triphala gently promotes internal cleansing to alleviate conditions stemming from stagnation and excess, while at the same time it improves digestion and nutrient absorption.

TRIKATU Trikatu, which means "three peppers" or "three pungents," is another triad of metabolism-enhancing natural botanicals made from long pepper (*Piper longum*), ginger (*Zingiber officinale*), and black pepper (*Piper nigrum*). A complementary formula to triphala, trikatu is traditionally used to support digestion and the overall gastric function, activating digestive enzymes and promoting rapid absorption of nutrients. Although it works primarily in the upper GI tract, it also lends a hand to the lower intestine. Trikatu's pungent qualities clear excess mucus from the body, which further aids digestion and supports respiratory function. Studies have shown that trikatu increases digestive absorption and assimilation by promoting rapid absorption through the intestines. It's also been shown to have anti-inflammatory effects and to reduce LDL ("bad") cholesterol, prevent the body from any allergic reactions, and help promote skin health. Because trikatu enhances digestion and the body's ability to prepare itself for food and the extraction of food's nutrients, this herbal remedy is ideal for supporting the *deepena* and *pachana* of stoking the body's agni.

As with triphala, trikatu is safe to use for a long period of time. It doesn't produce any side effects.

As I briefly noted earlier, I recommend that you take 500 mg twice daily of each supplement (for a total of 1,000 mg of each supplement daily) during the diet and consider making these a regular part of your routine even once your weight goals have been reached. Aim to take them on an empty stomach in between meals (about two hours before eating). On my website at www.hotbellydiet.com you'll find a list of brands to look for; although these supplements

> *Reminder: If you currently take any prescription medication, talk with your physician and share your plans before starting any supplement program. Although the ingredients of these supplements don't conflict with any drugs, it's always a good idea to check with your doctor and take into consideration any personal health challenges you have, along with your regular prescriptions. Because there are many manufacturers of supplements today, two formulas created for the same effect can have a different combination of ingredients as well as different dosages. To tailor the right supplements regimen to your body, start with your doctor and consider seeking the advice of a local naturopathic professional as well. If you go to www.hotbellydiet.com, you'll find further guidance in obtaining high-quality supplements as well as updated information on resources.*

may be new to you, they are highly accessible today both online and through retail outlets.

The first phase of the diet is very straightforward. Over the course of the next three days, you'll do the following:

> **Cut refined flours, processed carbohydrates, and some starches:** While you don't have to cut all carbs on this diet, prepare to change which carbs you consume by eliminating those that weaken your digestive fire. These include starchy

or sugary vegetables and any refined flours ("refined flour" has had the germ and bran removed and is typically called "white flour"). Starchy or sugary vegetables include corn, squash, white potatoes, sweet potatoes, yams, parsnips, beets, and turnips. (Don't panic: You can return to these after the 30 days.) Refined flour is processed—its core nutrients, like fiber, have been removed, and this creates a heavy stickiness that's hard on the body. It's also difficult to eliminate from the body, leading to incomplete evacuations (not enough fiber to move the bowel), so it sits and adds to the sludge, dampening your digestive fire. What's more, it can inhibit your body from extracting any nutrients at all from the food.

> **Cut "diet foods" such as products manufactured to be "low fat," "light," or "sugar free":** These products often contain ingredients that make up for that extracted fat and sugar and that dampen your digestive fire. I once treated a woman who was on a diet, but nothing was happening; she was eating gluten-free pizza every day with low-fat cheese. Little did she know that what she was consuming in these processed products was sabotaging her efforts. Gluten-free flours often contain potato flour and tapioca as a substitute, which is a processed ingredient worse than the real thing! And it can be more offensive to a gut that's sensitive to gluten, the protein normally found in wheat. What's more, any flour consumed with dairy (e.g., pizza dough and cheese) can create a digestive stickiness and heaviness.

> **Eliminate red meat and full-fat dairy:** Red meat takes a long time to digest, and dairy is a heavy food that can weaken your digestive fire and build mucus, which exacerbates ama. While I'll give you guidelines for reintroducing some red meat and full-fat dairy into your life during the maintenance phase, for now you'll avoid them.

> **Nix white sugar and artificial sweeteners, including those such as Truvía and Splenda:** While we like to think we're doing

ourselves good by replacing refined sugar with seminatural products like Truvía and Splenda (which are marketed as "made from nature"), these are processed chemicals in disguise. In Ayurveda, taste is an important component to the eating process. It signals the body and prepares it to digest the incoming food. Unfortunately, these processed sugar products can dupe the body: While it tastes sweet to you, the body cannot register the flavor and the sweetness cannot have an impact on satiety. So the body goes through a sluggish response, perpetuating that ama again. For a touch of sweetness, you can use honey or Stevia.

➤ **Reduce alcohol and liquid calories from sugary beverages:** The goal of this weaning process is to begin training the tongue to sense differently, to cut cravings, and to jump-start the weight-loss process. We need to train our body to learn the difference between how we feel at the sensorial level (i.e., the taste buds' and brain's interpretation of those sensations) and at the cellular, physical level. Many times, we enjoy foods on the tongue (and in our minds), but our body doesn't actually take pleasure in it. Or we can taste something we think we don't like, yet the body loves. The goal should be to create a cellular memory for what the mind *and* body both want. In Ayurvedic medicine, we call this the difference between *Shreyas*—what's eternally good for us and it doesn't matter whether your senses like them or not—and *Preyas,* or that which is purely sensorial and mental. In Phase 1, we're helping to establish the right balance between the Shreyas and the Preyas. In our eating life, we all reach for foods that might make us feel good in the short term, but may not necessarily be good for the body (e.g., sweets, pastries, fried foods), especially in the long term. And we may also opt for foods that we know are "healthy" (e.g., kale, fish, brown rice), but that our senses may not enjoy. So the goal is to transform Preyas—short-term choices based on the need for a pleasure fix—into Shreyas, sources of pleasure that are actually good for us, too. And that's the whole point of the Hot Belly Diet; it will train your body to love a way of eating you never before thought possible.

The Hot Belly Kitchen

In the days leading up to your new way of eating, you'll want to take an inventory of your kitchen and eliminate items that you'll no longer be consuming over the next month. The following is a list of products and ingredients to remove:

Refined flours, including baking and pastry flours and whole grain varieties

Bread

Noodles

White rice

Pastas

Pastries

Baked goods

Cereals

Corn

Yams, potatoes, sweet potatoes

Chips

Crackers

Cookies

Muffins

Pizza dough

Cakes

Doughnuts

Sugary snacks

Candy

Energy bars

Cow's milk

Cheese (including processed cheese spreads)

Ice cream/frozen yogurt/sherbet/sorbet

Jams/jellies/preserves

Ketchup and other condiments made with sugar

Fried foods

Sugar (white and brown), corn syrup, artificial sweeteners

Juices, sports/energy drinks, soft drinks/soda

Coffee

Diet foods (products labeled as "fat free," "low fat," "light")

"Gluten-free" foods: Because foods labeled as "gluten-free"
(or the following variations: "free of gluten"; "no gluten";
"without gluten") have become somewhat of a trend, it can
be difficult to distinguish between gluten-free foods that
are perfectly fine to consume and those that are not. Many
foods labeled "gluten-free" never contained gluten to begin
with (e.g., fruits, vegetables, eggs), but food manufacturers
are using this term on products that have been processed—
their gluten has been replaced by another ingredient such as

cornstarch, cornmeal, rice starch, potato starch, or tapioca starch, all of which can be equally as offensive. Although the FDA issued a regulation in August of 2013 to define the term for food labeling (the gluten limit for foods that carry any gluten-free label is less than twenty parts per million), it still leaves the burden on the manufacturers to comply and be accountable for using the claim truthfully.

Processed foods made with soy (i.e., soy cheese, soy burgers, soy hot dogs, soy nuggets, soy ice cream, soy yogurt)

Margarine, vegetable shortening, and any commercial brand of cooking oil (soybean, corn, cottonseed, canola, peanut, safflower, grape-seed, sunflower, rice bran, and wheat germ oils)

The specific ingredients you'll need to follow the Hot Belly Diet are straightforward. During Phase 1 and 2 you'll stick with primarily sattvic foods, which are fresh, pure, and vibrant. There are no chemicals, preservatives, pesticides, or fertilizers in these foods. The body easily digests sattvic foods, and their consumption prevents disease and promotes physical, mental, and spiritual health. While many of these foods have a rejuvenating effect on the body, they simultaneously have a calming effect on the mind. Most of these foods grow above the ground, where they are exposed to sunlight, making them lighter in nature than foods that mature below the ground.

Below is a list of what's allowable during the month-long diet. Wherever possible, go organic and local:

Almond milk (unsweetened)

Rice milk (unsweetened)

Protein powder made with whey isolate, hemp seeds, or brown rice (see www.hotbellydiet.com for brand recommendations)

Low-fat, low-sugar yogurt (Greek-style is best) or kefir

Mung beans

Lentils

Basmati, brown, and wild rice

Quinoa

Buckwheat

Oatmeal (avoid instant varieties; steel-cut is best)

Ground flaxseed

Shelled hemp seeds

Pumpkin seeds

Chia seeds

Raw sesame and sunflower seeds

Cashews, almonds, walnuts, pine nuts, and macadamia nuts

Fresh berries (all types; flash-frozen are fine)

Leafy greens: lettuce, spinach, kale, chard, collard greens, arugula, turnip greens, leeks, parsley

Cleansing vegetables: cauliflower, cabbage, broccoli, Brussels sprouts, carrots, artichokes, asparagus, onions, mushrooms, celery, bok choy, garlic, green beans, green peas, okra, scallions, cabbage, kale, fennel, radishes, watercress

Herbs and spices: You can use these liberally, but be sure to include cilantro, curry powder, cinnamon, nutmeg, and cardamom, as these are essential ingredients to some of the dishes designed to stir your agni and melt away the ama.

Lean proteins

Fish (opt for wild-caught when possible): salmon, black cod,
  mahimahi, grouper, herring, trout, flounder, sole, tilapia,
  shrimp, crab

Poultry: chicken, turkey

Eggs

Tofu

Tempeh

Cream-free soups, stews, and broths (so long as they are not
  loaded up with salt, sugar, and artificial ingredients)

Low-sugar fruits and vegetables: apples, berries, grapefruit,
  oranges, tangerines, peaches, nectarines, plums, kiwi, grapes,
  avocados, bell peppers, cucumbers, tomatoes, zucchini,
  eggplant, lemons, limes

Honey

Stevia

Extra-virgin olive oil and extra-virgin olive oil cooking spray

Ghee (a traditional Indian preparation of clarified butter that's
  readily found in supermarkets today)

Flaxseed oil

Sesame oil

Balsamic vinegar

A note about buying fresh produce: There's nothing more frus-
trating than splurging on fresh produce that wilts and begins to mold

the moment you get home. And you obviously don't want to run out and buy every possible fruit and vegetable listed above in one fell swoop. You'll want to plan which ones you intend to use in the coming days based on the meal plan and purchase them on an as-needed basis (unless you're going to stock up on frozen varieties). A few tips:

➤ Avoid bruised, dull-looking fruits and vegetables. Ask your grocer what just came in and what's local. Stick with what's in season if you're buying fresh produce. If you crave blueberries, but the "fresh" ones have been shipped from thousands of miles away, opt for flash-frozen ones instead. These will have been picked during the peak of their ripeness, thus retaining their nutrients.

➤ Brighter means better: The brighter the colors, the more nutrients the fruit or vegetable contains. When you have choices in color, such as buying various bell peppers or onions, choose an array. Different colors impart different nutrients.

➤ Limit the cooking of fruits and vegetables (steaming is best to preserve nutrients), and consume as many in the raw as possible.

➤ When cooking with frozen fruits and vegetables, don't thaw them out first, as this can allow microorganisms present in the food to multiply.

A note for vegetarians: I'm amused by people's erroneous belief that they need upwards of one hundred grams of protein a day. Vegetarians often ask me if they should worry about getting enough protein, and I reassure them that they obtain plenty from plant sources, legumes, dairy, and natural soy products such as tempeh and tofu. Nuts, seeds, and whole grains also contain protein. Most Americans get more than enough protein each day, and many could be getting too much from animal sources, such as meat, poultry, and eggs. Contrary to popular thinking, extra protein will not make you stronger or help you build more muscle. Protein is an essential component to any diet, but more doesn't mean better or healthier. When you're consuming too much of it, you're likely taking in more calories and fat than your body requires. According to the Centers for Disease Control and Prevention, we only need to get 10 to 35 percent of our day's calories from protein foods, which translates to about forty-six grams of protein for women, and fifty-six grams of protein for men. This is easy to consume when you consider the following: A small three-ounce piece of meat has about twenty-one grams of protein (if you eat a large eight-ounce piece of meat, it could contain more than fifty grams of protein); an eight-ounce container of yogurt has about eleven grams of protein; and one cup of dried beans has about sixteen grams of protein. On the Hot Belly Diet, you needn't worry about being deficient in protein. Far from it.

The First 3 Days of Meals

Here are examples of how you can create your first three days' worth of meals during Phase 1. Anything in *italics* will be found in the recipe section at the back of the book (Appendix A). By Day 3, you're nearly immersed in the protocol for the next several weeks. You can choose to follow this three-day menu exactly or create your own based on the above guidelines. Remember, at the very least, you should be avoiding processed and packaged foods, as well as refined flours, sugars, and heavy meals that entail red meat and full-fat dairy like cheese. Reduce your alcohol and coffee consumption as much as possible, if not entirely, and swap all other beverages such as sodas and fruit drinks with the daily drink prescribed (see page 102). Make lunch your biggest meal of the day. No snacking. If you find it hard to avoid nibbling on something in between meals, then take a ten- to twenty-minute walk around the block and drink warm water. Your craving will go away. If you truly cannot nix the urge to chew on something, try some sugar-free gum. Be done with dinner before 7:00 p.m.

The Daily Drink

Every day throughout this program from 8:00 a.m. to 4:00 p.m., you'll sip a green tea blend that can easily be made in the morning and placed in a stainless steel thermos to last the entire day. Start drinking this tea during the Prepare Phase so you get used to this practice, which you may want to continue after the month-long diet. My wish is for you to adopt the habit of drinking hot, hydrating liquids daily. This delicious "live detox" includes a blend of cumin, coriander, fennel seeds, fresh ginger, and lemon juice, with the green tea brew as the base. It will stimulate your digestive juices and rev your metabolism, for the compounds in the brew help to burn fat. It also keeps you hydrated, a key factor in maintaining that healthy agni to absorb nutrients properly and in "stirring the pot" of your digestive processes. Here's how to make the green tea blend:

> In 1 quart of water over medium-high heat, add a teaspoonful each of whole fennel, coriander, and cumin seeds. Add a half teaspoon of freshly grated ginger and then bring the mixture to a boil with one tea bag of organic green tea. Strain it into a stainless steel thermos and squirt in the juice from half a lemon. If you're sensitive to caffeine, opt for caffeine-free green tea. For those short on time, you can look for green teas in the market that contain lemon and ginger. Just be sure they don't also contain other additives like sugar and chemicals.

When you want to switch to a caffeine-free drink or avoid green tea, you can also choose to sip plain hot water with a squeeze of lemon and a slice of fresh ginger, or try herbal teas.

Day 1

➤ Breakfast: 2 eggs scrambled with 2 cleansing vegetables (see page 98) of your choice, or a bowl (one serving) of steel-cut oatmeal made with water and 1 tablespoon ground flaxseed,

topped with a small handful of raw walnuts or almonds and
¼ cup fresh berries

➤ Lunch: 3 to 4 ounces grilled fish, tofu, or tempeh with
steamed cleansing vegetables (see page 98) and ½ cup brown
rice + 1 piece of whole fruit as dessert.

➤ Dinner: Salad greens with 3 ounces of lean poultry (chicken or
turkey), tofu, or tempeh

Day 2

➤ Breakfast: 1 cup low-fat yogurt topped with a small handful of
raw walnuts, fresh berries, and a drizzle of honey (optional)

➤ Lunch: 4 ounces poached salmon with a side salad dressed
with olive oil vinaigrette + 1 piece of whole fruit as dessert

➤ Dinner: A bowl of meat-free soup, such as lentil, broccoli, or
tomato

Day 3

➤ Breakfast: *Superfood Smoothie*

➤ Lunch: *Midday Khichadi* + 1 piece of whole fruit as dessert

➤ Dinner: *Grilled Vegetables with Miso Sauce* over a bed of
steamed jasmine rice

Don't forget to use the Hunger Meter (page 79) to check in with
yourself and fine-tune your portions and eating experience. Remember, eating is just one-fifth of your "consumption." You can go a lot
longer without actual food than without breath or water. We place
so much importance on calories today that we forget how to enjoy
our meals and treat food as just one small source of vital energy. No
other science talks about perceiving the world through your senses
and creating a body out of all that. Your perception of the world—
and of yourself—is from what you take in, and how you metabolize
not just calories, but all of your experiences.

CHAPTER 5

Phase 2: Accelerate

DAYS 4–26

Diet is what you take in from any field of perception, from any mode of intellect.

—UPANISHADS (SACRED VEDIC TEXTS)

ere comes the main part of the diet. Now that you've gained an enormous amount of information and inspiration from the previous chapters, it's time to put it all to the test. But I've made this really easy: You won't have to do any math or second-guessing as to what exactly you are supposed to eat during the next 21 days. I will lay out every single meal and provide a few optional guidelines to follow should you need to make any personal modifications. Such modifications could be for:

➤ Someone who is carb-sensitive per the questionnaire in Chapter 2.
➤ Someone who doesn't like the taste of a particular ingredient used in preparing khichadi. (Despite the reliance on this meal during the Accelerate Phase, I offer a variety of different versions by rotating the grains and vegetables. I will explain how you can customize the recipes to your unique preferences. You can't get bored on this diet!)

➤ Someone who requires more calories in the form of protein due to physical needs.

➤ Someone who doesn't enjoy shakes and wants more substantial food in place of one.

It's easy to remember what to eat during Phase 2. A typical day looks like the following:

➤ Breakfast: Superfood Smoothie (see below); or a bowl (one serving) of steel-cut oatmeal made with water and 1 tablespoon ground flaxseed, topped with a small handful of raw walnuts or almonds and ¼ cup fresh berries; or an egg-veggie scramble made with 2 eggs plus 1 egg white and leafy greens, bell peppers, and mushrooms.

➤ Lunch: Midday Khichadi (page 106)

➤ Dinner: Suppertime Khichadi (page 108); or Superfood Smoothie (below); or a bowl of meat-free, non-creamy soup with a side of steamed cleansing vegetables (see page 98).

SUPERFOOD SMOOTHIE

Serves 1

⅔ cup unsweetened organic almond milk or rice milk (no soy milk)

⅔ cup water

2 scoops protein powder in the form of whey isolate, hemp seed protein powder, or brown rice protein powder (a list of brands to look for can be found at www.hotbellydiet .com; the product will include the scoop for measuring)

1 tablespoon whole flaxseed, shelled hemp seeds, or raw sunflower seeds, and a small handful of blueberries, raspberries, or blackberries

Pinch of cinnamon, pinch of nutmeg, and/or pinch of cardamom powder (choose two of these three)

Mix all the ingredients in a blender.

Variation: For added sweetness, add 1 teaspoon of unheated raw honey or Stevia. Those who don't want to use almond or rice milk can opt for ¼ cup yogurt (1% fat Greek-style) or ¼ cup kefir and 1 cup water instead.

Note: Play with different berries, types of milk, flavors of protein, and types of seeds on a daily basis. For those who need more for breakfast, add a hard-boiled egg.

MIDDAY KHICHADI

Serves 1

¼ cup basmati rice or buckwheat (use organic)

½ cup split mung beans (use organic)

2 ½ cups water

2 teaspoons olive oil

1 ½ teaspoons curry powder

Salt

3 to 4 stems and leaves of fresh cilantro, finely chopped

1 cup finely chopped cleansing vegetables (see page 98)

1 tablespoon raw, unsalted seeds of your choice (see options, page 98)

2 tablespoons chopped raw nuts of your choice (see options, page 98)

Rinse the rice and beans. In a medium pot, combine the water, rice, and beans and bring to a boil. Reduce the heat to a low boil and continue cooking for 20 to 30 minutes. Add the olive oil, curry powder, and salt while cooking. Stir well in between.

At the end, add the cilantro, vegetables, seeds, and nuts. Stir well and serve hot.

Note: On my website, you'll find resources for buying pre-made khichadi packets that require as little preparation as possible. All of these ingredients can readily be found in today's grocery stores. If you're in a rush, khichadi can be prepared within minutes in the morning and taken with you for lunch. Here's how: Mix all the ingredients into boiling water for a couple of minutes, then transfer to a wide-mouth thermos and close the lid. Over the next couple of hours, the mixture will slow-cook to perfection so your lunch is ready by midday. Rotate which leafy greens and vegetables you use so you don't eat the same style of khichadi twice in a row.

Variation for carb-sensitive individuals: If you scored high on the carb quiz in Chapter 2, then make the khichadi with just the mung beans and skip the rice or buckwheat. So use ¾ cup mung beans; and if that doesn't work, then go lean and green. Or try sprouting your green mung beans and add them to a salad. This can be done by washing whole mung beans, soaking them overnight in room-temperature water, then straining them and wrapping them in cheesecloth the next day. The beans will have sprouted by the evening. When you sprout your grains, you positively change their chemical makeup by changing the composition of the starch molecules, converting them into vegetable sugars. Such a change means the body recognizes and digests sprouted grains as a vegetable, and the enzymes created during the sprouting process are known to aid digestion. Moreover, the process increases the grain's vitamin content while neutralizing carcinogens and enzyme inhibitors, as well as an acid that inhibits absorption of calcium, magnesium, iron, copper, and zinc. Once you've sprouted your beans, store them in an airtight glass jar in your kitchen at room temperature and consume them within four days.

"But I don't like curry. What can I do?" If you don't enjoy the taste curry powder imparts, try ground cumin, coriander, and black pepper.

"I need something more substantial at lunch. Can I skip the khichadi and do something else for lunch?" Certainly. One of the most important guidelines, however, is to keep dinner as light as possible

and make lunch your most important meal of the day. If you prefer, prepare a mixed green salad for lunch with a three- to four-ounce portion of lean protein such as fish, chicken, turkey, or tofu. Dress with a simple balsamic vinegar and a drizzle of olive oil or flaxseed oil with a squeeze of lemon (no creamy or packaged dressings). Serve with a side of a half cup of brown rice. Or, in lieu of the salad greens with your protein, steam a blend of cleansing vegetables (see page 98). Another option is to add a *Lassi* to your lunch, which is a traditional Indian drink made by blending fresh yogurt with room temperature water. Yogurt by itself can clog the channels of the digestive system, including elimination, but once it is transformed into a Lassi, it actually aids digestion. When you thin yogurt with water, you change the molecular structure so it's more easily assimilated in the body. You can drink either Sweet Lassi or Salty (Digestive) Lassi before or with lunch. (Both recipes are in Appendix A.)

Note: If you choose something other than khichadi at lunch, be sure to have khichadi for dinner, then. During the Accelerate Phase, the goal is to have at least one serving of khichadi a day, either at lunch or dinner.

SUPPERTIME KHICHADI

Serves 1

At dinner, aim to prepare a soupier khichadi by replacing the cleansing vegetables (see page 98) with your choice of 1 cup finely chopped leafy greens: lettuce, spinach, kale, chard, collard greens, arugula, turnip greens, leeks, and parsley. Also, replace the rice or buckwheat with ¼ cup quinoa, and skip the nuts. For those who need more than just this, you can also have a 1-cup side of steamed cleansing vegetables of your choice. I realize that many of you are used to eating a much larger dinner, and having a protein-rich plate with meat, fish, or poultry and a side of rice or potatoes. Once you lighten up your evening meal to something very simple to digest (khichadi, soup, or a smoothie), you'll notice a remarkable difference in your sleep quality that night and your energy the next day. Such a light meal further creates a mini twelve-hour fast that goes from lunch to lunch every day.

Dessert: For those who need a sweet ending to their day, you've got a few options. One is to have a serving of 70 percent dark chocolate, or a serving of fresh fruit or fruit in the form of dates, figs, dried apricots, or raisins.

Don't Forget to Drink

Drink your hot green tea blend (see page 102) throughout the day until about 4 p.m., after which you can switch to plain hot water with lemon and ginger, or herbal teas. Hot beverages, especially those infused with lemon and ginger, are incredibly good for digestion and stirring agni. Look for organic teas in the market that contain lemon and ginger or simply prepare your own using thick slices of fresh ginger and wedges of lemon.

Walk After Each Meal

Everyone knows that exercise is good for us (and our waistlines). But not everyone realizes that exercise needn't entail training for a marathon or sweating it out for an hour on a machine in the gym. In Chapter 7, I'll be taking you behind the scenes of why starting a yoga routine can complement the Hot Belly Diet perfectly and provide a wonderful foundation for your future health beyond the core phase of the diet. It's best to avoid rigorous physical activity (e.g., anything that gets your heart rate pumping hard) while your body is purging during Phase 2, especially if you've been sedentary, but you should aim to walk soon after every meal for a minimum of twenty minutes, as this will encourage your body's flow of metabolic hormones and substances that help support your digestive health and agni. If you're accustomed to physical exercise, then by all means keep up with your routine during the diet so long as you feel strong and able. But you don't need to jump immediately into a high-intensity workout regimen during this diet.

Be Mindful as You Eat

Our eating experience is just as important as *what* we're eating. If we're having an argument with someone over the dinner table, our body detects the distress and sends chemical messages that inhibit the creation of ojas.

Because ojas is the by-product of all the signals our body receives, it's imperative that we create a nurturing atmosphere while we eat, paying attention to all of the senses—taste, sound, sight, touch, and smell. Here are a few tips for making your body happy while you eat:

➤ Eat in a settled, quiet, comfortable atmosphere. Such a setting promotes ideal digestion. Approach your eating sessions as sacred times to relax and recharge rather than an obligation on your to-do list. Savor the food itself, focusing on its flavors and textures.

➤ Don't eat when you're upset, emotional, or angry. When you eat while seething from negative emotions, you can disrupt your body's natural, rhythmic flow of a healthy digestion. The tightening of muscles and the release of stress hormones will directly sabotage your body's digestive powers, including its ability to absorb nutrients. Avoid heated discussions and arguments while eating, too. If necessary, delay eating until you've calmed down. Emotionally heightened states can also be problematic even if they are positive, so if you find yourself excessively excited for some reason, postpone eating until your emotions have normalized. This doesn't mean you avoid eating while laughing with friends, but learn to check in with yourself to assess whether or not it's a good idea to give yourself more time to wind down before eating.

➤ Always sit down to eat in a place free of distractions such as the TV, the computer, and even reading material. (And, it goes without saying, avoid driving while eating!) I realize that we live in an age where "on-the-go" eating is the norm. But sitting down has enormous effects on the digestive system. When you sit during a meal, you help the body relax and allow the digestive process to take place effortlessly. When you eat while standing or walking, digestion requires more energy (and if it's not readily available, you will cramp up).

➤ Eat on a regular schedule. Have breakfast, lunch, and dinner at roughly the same time daily. If this requires that you keep an alarm clock for a week so you train your body to eat at specific times that maintain a similar pattern, do so. The body is an amazing but delicate piece of machinery. Attuning your body's innate clock with the natural rhythms of nature is one of the fundamental aims of Ayurveda. It's not arbitrary that lunchtime—the biggest meal of the day—coincides with midday, as this is when the sun is highest in the sky and your agni is strongest. When you eat in accordance with the rhythms of nature, you support your body's underlying, natural makeup. By eating on a consistent, regular schedule, you ensure that your body stays maximally nourished and energized while also keeping cravings at bay and avoiding overeating.

➤ Listen to your body's hunger and respond to it. Only eat when you're hungry, and stop when you reach a point of comfort. You want to feel satisfied but not full. If you stuff your stomach with too much food, there's not enough room for the digestive process to take place. Eating when you're not hungry is the equivalent of putting too much wood on the fire; the digestive fire will be snuffed out. This leads to incomplete digestion and assimilation of nutrients, which in turn encourages the build-up of ama. So don't let yourself go over that edge after which you wish you hadn't had that "last bite" or taken that last helping. Remember, the stomach expands as we eat, but it can take time for our brains to receive the signal that we've had enough. Pause throughout your meal to assess where you are on the Hunger Meter (page 79), then proceed accordingly. This may sound so simple and straightforward, but plenty of people struggle daily to resist eating when they aren't even hungry.

➤ Respect the mini-fast in between meals. It usually takes three to six hours to digest a meal (everyone will be different in this department). A pitta person will digest food faster than a kapha person, for example. If you want to avoid dousing the digestive fire, you need to allow the digestive system ample time to do its work. So, how do you know it's time to eat again? It's when you feel hungry and have a sense of lightness in your belly. Many people don't understand what it feels like to experience genuine hunger because they have extreme cycles of blood-sugar imbalances that mask their sense of true hunger. There's a difference between blood sugar crashes and true hunger, and my wish for you on this diet is that you begin to sense the latter rather than the former. The last time you may have felt real hunger may have occurred following an illness during which you lost your appetite. But as your body healed, your appetite returned and you responded to it.

➤ Take time to finish your meal. Don't gulp down your food or eat too slowly. A meal should take twenty to thirty minutes to finish. Chew your food thoroughly so that your body can properly digest and assimilate that food. Digestion actually starts in the mouth as you break down food particles into usable parts for the stomach to handle. It's no joke we digest more than 40 percent of complex carbohydrates during the process of chewing alone. Which is why Ayurveda respects chewing as an important part of any weight-loss program. Why else would we be equipped with sharp teeth and saliva that's filled with enzymes to break down food on the spot? When you chew your food thoroughly, you will automatically regulate your eating pace while at the same time unleash the flavors of the food itself.

➤ Rest briefly after each meal. While it's a good idea to move the body after a meal, hence my recommendation to walk for twenty minutes or so, do take a couple of minutes to relax and enjoy the feeling of satiety once you're done eating. Then you can get up and go.

In Chapter 9, you'll find a host of tips for optimizing your eating experiences beyond Phase 2.

Closing Cleanse

On the last day of the Accelerate Phase, you can opt to do the castor oil cleanse once more or stick with liquids all day (juices, teas, and brothy soups). This can further accelerate your results and set the tone for Phase 3.

CHAPTER 6

Phase 3: Transform

DAYS 27–30 AND BEYOND

Let noble thoughts come to us from every side.

—THE RIG VEDA, A COLLECTION OF HYMNS
COMPOSED IN THE SECOND MILLENNIUM BC

Congratulations. You've been on the Hot Belly Diet now for three weeks and should be feeling different from the way you did three weeks ago. Are your clothes looser? Do you feel lighter, more energetic, able to accomplish more throughout the day? Are symptoms that were once chronic fading or vanishing? Are you getting restful sleep nightly? Does your skin look younger? Do you have fewer cravings? Is your mood and overall attitude better? I hope so, and if the transformation has been slow or subtle, don't panic. This chapter will help you reach your goal.

Welcome to the Transform Phase. This is the "rest of your life" phase, as well as the one that guides you through the transition from the core diet phase to one in which you feel in control of your eating habits and can support radiant health and your ideal weight for the long run. This is where you learn how to keep your weight loss going and maintain your goal weight for life. The Accelerate Phase got your weight loss revving in high gear by detoxifying the system, eradicating impurities and blockages, and creating the flow and fire necessary to keep the body burning and building healthy tissues. Just because you're leaving the core diet phase and reintroducing foods you love doesn't mean the weight loss stops! Much to the contrary, this is where weight loss can really take off. You've done the hard work of resetting—rekindling—your metabolism. It's now a matter of keeping your engine burning brightly.

I will first guide you step-by-step through the process of leaving the Accelerate Phase and reintroducing certain foods over the next four days. Now is the time to start adding more options back into your diet and to learn how to eat whatever you want (but not as much as you want) without worrying about your choices sabotaging your efforts or reversing your gains. You'll then be able to consider alcohol, coffee, red meat, a wider selection of carbs, including starchy vegetables, and more desserts from Day 31 onward. Once I outline your Transform Phase parameters, I will offer all the practical tools you need to live up to the main principles of the Hot Belly Diet in your life while enjoying a much more expansive array of foods.

As you're already aware of by now, Ayurveda endorses a balanced diet that nurtures not only the body, but also the mind, sense, and spirit. Food, after all, is a source of energy and strength. It's sustenance and radiance. Ayurvedic nutrition is intimately tied to the three doshas and takes into account the unique dietary requirements of every individual. Eating in accordance with your constitutional makeup promotes balance, while eating dosha-aggravating foods creates imbalances. The very concept that "food is medicine" is special to Ayurveda. Food is the primary preventive tool in Ayurveda, as well as the first step in bringing the mind and body back into balance. Although we often say, "You are what you eat," Ayurveda would modify that to say, "You are what, how, when, and why you eat." Your well-being results not only from the types of foods you eat, but also from your state of mind, the environment, the time of day, and the season in which you consume them.

Westerners like to think of food as being separate from the body, much like a car uses gas to fuel up and make it go. But food itself is an energetic force just like the body, so we cannot detach ourselves from the food we eat. This energy—or prana—of food not only nourishes each cell on a physical and biological level, but also replenishes our entire life force.

We also tend to think of food in the West as comprising different nutritional qualities. For example, we have classes of foods such as carbohydrates, fats, and proteins, each of which can be further classified by how much energy or how many calories per gram they contain. Ayurveda similarly classifies foods in relation to their energetic qualities and effects on the doshas, the digestion, and the mind. As you already know by now, imbalances within the doshas lead to improper digestion that in turn can trigger future illness. Ayurvedic nutrition incorporates the mental effects of nutrition as well, respecting the fact that food influences the qualities of the mind. Take, for instance, the emotions we can feel upon eating a certain food, such as spicy food's ability to make us mad and animated. What's more, Ayurveda recognizes that we process food mentally in the form of sensory impressions, thoughts, and emotions. Big meals, for example, can lead to indigestion and heartburn and ultimately disharmony of the mind—what we'd call "mental indigestion."

What's inviting about an Ayurvedic approach to diet is that it doesn't entail a rigid set of one-plan-fits-all guidelines. It offers a universal system of nutrition that teaches us how to eat in accordance with our individual dosha. All foods can be evaluated within an Ayurvedic framework; Ayurvedic nutrition will never live up to today's fad diets that label certain foods as "good" or "bad." Instead, it places the greatest emphasis on your own instinctive ability to feed yourself healthfully.

That said, it helps to have some kind of rule book for implementing an Ayurvedic approach to your lifestyle, and for figuring out exactly which kind of dietary protocol will work for you and your dosha. By now you've gotten a head start in resetting your body back to its natural, factory-installed programming and can better get in touch with your internal machinery to proceed. Much of the Ayurvedic wisdom about nutrition is right there on your tongue. The sense of taste should be a natural guide toward proper nutrition. After all, we've always relied largely on our taste buds to tell us what's healthy versus what's toxic (only in recent times has food engineering confused our innate instincts about taste and nutrition). Our taste buds do more than just provide us a flavor; they begin the process of breaking down food so it can be used as energy by the body.

For this very reason, Ayurveda identifies six tastes by which all foods can be categorized: sweet, salty, sour, bitter, pungent (i.e., hot and spicy, like a chili pepper), and astringent (i.e., like leafy greens). And, similar to the body's physical and energetic makeup, the six tastes are combinations of the five elements (space, air, fire, water, and earth). Nutritional balance, then, is found within the six tastes, and we should experience all six tastes in our eating habits. From a modern nutritional perspective, the six tastes satisfy each of the major dietary building blocks: By incorporating the six tastes into each meal, we get a complete package of nutrition. We also achieve two big goals:

1. As those different taste buds get lit up by the various tastes, they each have unique connections with the digestive juices and enzymes in the gut. When all are stimulated properly, the juices flow completely. The six tastes essentially stimulate the proper sequence of digestion; they can be thought of as essential links in a complex digestive chain. Conversely, if you don't have all the juices flowing, you become vulnerable to the buildup of sludge on the tongue and then you cannot taste completely, which starts a vicious cycle that ends up with systemic ama.

2. Remember that everyone contains all three doshas at their core. That's why including all six tastes in a meal is the most important way to nourish each dosha (and thus every person) at a fundamental level. Most of us have a strong secondary dosha,

which greatly expands the number of foods that help balance our overall body.

It's important to differentiate between easy-to-digest tastes (and, hence, foods that are easy to digest) and those that demand more energy (i.e., they are heavier and take longer to digest). The Hot Belly Diet does this for you, and the dietary recommendations in this phase further help you to achieve this balance of tastes. I'll also offer ideas on tailoring your protocol to your dominant dosha, which you figured out in Chapter 3.

Note that our epidemic of nutritional imbalance is greatly linked to our cultural bias toward the first two flavors: sweet and salty. Excess consumption of sweet and salty tastes is an overwhelming contributing factor to obesity, high blood pressure, diabetes, and heart disease. Fast- and processed-food manufacturers know the power of these two tastes, which is why they incorporate as much of these into their products as possible, crowding out the room for the other flavors. But once you gain an appreciation for all six tastes in a single meal and know how to spot and correct imbalances, you'll automatically find yourself moving away from these nutritional deserts in favor of nutrient-dense foods that harmonize with your body. In fact, the taste buds regenerate every 10 to 14 days. If you've been following the Hot Belly Diet already for this long, then your taste buds have reset. This allows you to take charge of your diet by developing a palate for all six flavors. And that's exactly what this phase is designed to do.

PHASE 3 PROTOCOL The eating plan for the next four days couldn't be simpler: You will change just *one* meal. So, for instance, you'll keep the same plan for lunch and dinner as you did during Phase 2, but you'll change your breakfast; or you'll change your dinner but maintain the same breakfast and lunch. This is where you can begin to experiment with new recipes and go beyond just limiting your daily fare to the options given in Phase 2. Three rules, however, will help you stay on track:

➤ Eat a bowl of khichadi once a day as a meal.
➤ Make lunch your heartiest meal of the day. This can mean a bowl of khichadi with a side of lean protein such as grilled chicken, fish, or tofu or a bed of leafy greens. (Aim for hot, non-creamy soups or Suppertime Khichadi [page 108] at dinner.)
➤ Continue to avoid foods that are not listed on page 97–99. I'll teach you how to incorporate foods like red meat, alcohol, full-fat dairy like cheese, flours, and sugars back into your diet once you've crossed the one-month threshold.

Don't get too fancy during these four days. You'll stick with foods that are light and easy to digest, such as steamed or stir-fried vegetables, soups, curries, stews, broths, combinations of different beans and lentils, lean animal protein in small quantities such as turkey, chicken, and fish, and tofu. And you'll continue to prepare khichadi daily, drink hot liquids throughout the day, and keep your evening meal as light as possible. For dessert, use the same options as before (one serving of dark chocolate or a serving of fruit in the form of dates, figs, dried apricots, or raisins).

Here is a four-day sample menu plan that you can use as your guideline. You can follow this exactly or create your own within the given parameters. You'll find the recipes for any meals in italics in Appendix A.

Morning Drink

Each day when you get up, drink a cup of warm water with a squeeze of lemon and a slice of fresh ginger. This will stimulate your digestive process and stir your agni. Prepare your green tea blend (see page 102) as part of your morning routine. You'll want to sip this metabolism booster throughout the day, as you did during the previous phases.

Day 27

➤ Breakfast: Veggie scramble with 2 whole eggs and 1 egg white and mushrooms and bell peppers or a bowl of oatmeal or a smoothie

➤ Lunch: *Midday Khichadi* + 1 side of lean protein + 1 piece of whole fruit as dessert (optional)

➤ Dinner: *Asparagus Soup*

Day 28:

➤ Breakfast: *Coconut-Cucumber Smoothie* + 1 hard-boiled egg (optional)

➤ Lunch: 3 ounces of poached salmon seasoned with fresh dill and lemon + ½ cup brown rice + stir-fried vegetables + 1 piece of whole fresh fruit as dessert (optional)

➤ Dinner: *Suppertime Khichadi*

Day 29:

➤ Breakfast: *Yogurt Parfait with Low-Fat Granola*

➤ Lunch: 3 to 4 ounces of lean protein of choice over *Wild Rice Salad with Fennel* + 1 piece of whole fresh fruit as dessert (optional)

➤ Dinner: *Pumpkin Soup* + 1 cup steamed cleansing vegetables (see page 98)

Day 30:

➤ Breakfast: *Hot Quinoa Cereal with Warm Spiced Milk*

➤ Lunch: *Midday Khichadi* + 1 piece of whole fresh fruit as dessert (optional)

➤ Dinner: *Kale and Mandarin Salad* + 1 cup brothy soup

Life After the 30-Day Plan: Cultivating a Healthy Tongue

Now that you've spent the past month limiting your diet to certain foods that have reprogrammed your metabolism and taste buds, it is time to begin adding more variety back and not worrying about the occasional slip (i.e., your birthday cake, cocktails at a party, your best friend's wedding weekend) derailing your good intentions and dietary ideals. At this point, you can consider bringing back foods that we had "de-listed" earlier, such as bread, cheese, red meat, alcohol, and sweets. Here's how, alongside a few other tips to consider.

Mindful Moderation

Although foods high in sugar, fat, and salt, and heavy meals that include red meat, starchy vegetables (e.g., potatoes), full-fat dairy, and alcohol can weaken your digestive fire, that doesn't mean you have to exclude them for the rest of your life. Some of these ingredients can actually assist your digestive fire so long as you don't consume them in excess. But these days, too many of us overindulge, turning a benefit into a digestive liability. Indeed, there's something to be said for too much of a good thing.

So you just have to learn how to balance your vices with your virtues—that is to say, the inherently virtuous foods with those that can lead to imbalances when over-consumed. And no two people will be the same in this department. A kapha person, for instance, might be able to devour a bucket of movie popcorn and feel great, while a vata type will quickly feel bloated and gassy. Ayurveda aims not to generalize food and food rules. Banning all sugars, for example, under the thinking that all sugar is bad, is not a useful goal. There's a difference between refined sugars and natural ones that can help balance some people out. And despite the popular wisdom of the day, even our most vilified vices in the modern era can have beneficial qualities when consumed smartly. To this end, let me offer some advice.

> Continue to prepare and consume khichadi three to four times a week as well as drinking hot water throughout the day (three to four cups a day with ginger and lemon).

> Stick to making lunch your main meal most of the time.

> Prepare lighter dinners than usual twice a week (e.g., soups, smoothies, or khichadi), and skip breakfast the next morning.

> Have plenty of steamed or stir-fried cleansing vegetables (see page 98) daily. You can add starchy and sugary vegetables back into your diet in moderation (two to three times per week).

> Use fruit, nuts, and seeds, and low-fat yogurt as a snack *if necessary*. Avoid snacking in general, but I realize that sometimes that's not always possible or practical. Keep in mind, however, that the more you can avoid snacking, the more you can stabilize blood sugar.

> Eggs are a great source of lean, digestible protein. Aim for 4 to 6 eggs per week.

> Avoid eating meat twice in the same day.

> If you're a meat eater, limit red meat to once weekly, and choose lean cuts of organic, grass-fed beef. To increase the digestibility of red meat, cook it with digestive herbs and spices such as cumin, fennel, garlic, and salt. Avoid buying meat packaged in foam or sealed with plastic wrap, due to potential toxicity.

> Consume white protein (e.g., chicken, turkey, tofu) two to three times weekly.

> Consume fish (wild-caught) two to three times weekly.

> Minimize flours and choose multigrain or sprouted-wheat breads.

- Choose multigrain rice or buckwheat pastas and noodles over white varieties.
- Eat cheese in moderation. Opt for aged hard cheese or soft cheese such as goat and cottage cheese.
- Buy organic cow's milk if you drink milk or use it in recipes. Also don't forget to try milks made from natural soy, nuts, and rice, and goat's milk.
- Severely limit fried, processed, packaged, and sugary foods and sweets.
- Enjoy freshly prepared condiments such as chutneys and spice mixtures.
- Favor natural sweeteners such as raw sugar, honey, and maple syrup rather than white table sugar and anything with corn syrup.
- Consume alcohol and coffee in moderation. This means one cup of coffee a day—before 2:00 p.m. (preferably without added sugar or milk); and a glass of wine with dinner (preferably red).
- If you have a big dinner, then skip breakfast the next morning and wait until you're hungry (don't have a banquet dinner and then a buffet breakfast).
- Avoid weekend binges. If you overindulge, have a soupy light dinner on Sunday night and skip breakfast Monday morning.

Other Items to Use in Moderation

Microwave Ovens: Although some research has shown that microwave cooking, which rapidly cooks food mostly by heating the water molecules, can alter the molecular structure of food, microwaves are not "dangerous" by any measure. And alarmist claims that they can promote harmful changes in blood composition are based on unreliable, suspect studies. The issue, however, is that rarely do these appliances that make cooking and reheating fast and convenient support eating live, vibrant foods that work in synch with your digestive system. So avoid them if you can. Engage in the cooking process as much as possible. By the same token, avoid leftovers (especially ones you have to microwave!). Leftover, instant, and precooked foods are as far from the Hot Belly Diet as you can get.

Deep Freeze: Defrosted foods begin to decompose quickly, often becoming dry, colorless, flavorless, and odorous in a short time period. Their life force has been compromised. With the exception of flash-frozen fruits and vegetables, avoid cooking with foods that come out of the freezer. Instead, aim for eating freshly prepared foods. In addition, the longer a food stays in the refrigerator, the more lifeless it becomes.

Food Combinations to Avoid

Cheese in your oatmeal? Peanut butter on your eggs? Certain foods just don't go together. But it's not just about the taste experience. Certain food combinations can stir the proverbial ama pot and create unwanted by-products in the gut. You wouldn't think to make a breakfast drink that's equal parts milk and OJ, but if we drink these two beverages separately at the same meal (a common American habit), they can curdle in our stomachs and make digestion difficult. Ayurveda identifies a few food combinations that you would do well to avoid. Some of these will surprise you if you've gotten used to eating these combinations, many of which relate to dairy products. If you've eaten these combinations without any problems whatsoever in the past, it's possible that your body has gotten used to them and you cannot sense any symptoms such as indigestion or cramping. But that doesn't mean you're home free. These combinations could be quietly affecting you just by disrupting optimal absorption of nutrients, encouraging intestinal sludge, and triggering silent inflammatory pathways. You could benefit mightily from avoiding them in the future. Here they are:

- Milk in combination with meat, fish, eggs, bananas, yogurt, or sour fruits
- Yogurt with milk, eggs, hot drinks, cheese, fish, tomatoes, potatoes, eggplant, or lemons
- Eggs with milk, meat, fish, yogurt, cheese, fruit, or beans
- Fresh fruits with any other foods, since many create sour juices or "wines" in the stomach. Cooked fruits are easier to digest with other foods. Avoid fresh, whole fruit as a dessert after meals, as the energy of fruits should not be exposed to hot, digestive acids.

Avoid Cold and Carbonated Drinks with Meals

Drinking cold fluids directly inhibits agni. Cold drinks shock the digestive system, and carbonated drinks create excess gas. Aim to stick with drinking hot liquids such as warm water or tea, and if possible, drink a glass of room-temperature water an hour after eating.

Balance Your Dosha

The longer you stay on the Hot Belly Diet, the closer you'll get to being in tune with your underlying nature. This will compel you to seek foods with balancing tastes while avoiding those that irritate your digestive system. Contrary to other diets, Ayurveda favors experimental learning over strict adherence to rules. Only then can you establish what works for you and your individual constitution. As you develop your awareness for your true dietary needs (including likes and dislikes), you'll effortlessly discover how to fine-tune your health through food.

Below are some guidelines to consider when tweaking your diet to your dominant dosha:

General Dietary Tips for Vata

Eat foods with sweet, sour, and salty tastes and avoid those that are bitter, pungent, and/or astringent.

Make a balanced breakfast each morning.

Don't eat when upset, nervous, or anxious.

Take note of any signs of poor digestion (e.g., gas, bloating, diarrhea, constipation).

Limit white sugar and caffeine.

Favor heavier whole grains such as rice, quinoa, and oats, as well as heavier fruits such as mangoes, bananas, dates, oranges, grapes, and grapefruit.

Enjoy heavy, moist vegetables such as squash and sweet potatoes, while limiting nightshades (tomatoes and eggplant).

Watch out for digestive issues with cow's milk and hard cheeses.

General Dietary Tips for Pitta

Eat foods with sweet, bitter, and astringent tastes and avoid those that are salty, sour, and/or pungent.

Make a balanced breakfast and have an early lunch.

Limit refined sugar, alcohol, and caffeine.

Don't conduct business while eating.

Choose basmati rice, quinoa, and whole grain pastas over corn, rye, and buckwheat.

Limit sour and heating vegetables such as mustard greens, tomatoes, radishes, garlic, and eggplant.

Watch out for peanuts, cashews, pistachios, and salted nuts.

Favor white meats and fish over red meats.

General Dietary Tips for Kapha

Eat foods with bitter, pungent, and astringent tastes, and avoid those that are sweet, sour, and/or salty.

Watch portions.

Make a light breakfast and a light evening meal.

Avoid frequent snacking and late-night eating.

Limit white sugar and greasy foods.

Drink warm beverages.

Enjoy toasted whole grain and sprouted-wheat breads and popped grains such as corn and amaranth.

Eat light fruits such as apples, pears, and cranberries, and dried fruit, and limit heavy fruits such as pineapple, oranges, melon, and bananas.

Eat a wide spectrum of produce, but limit avocados, sweet potatoes, and tomatoes.

Go for pumpkin seeds and sunflower seeds instead of coconut, almonds, sesame seeds, peanuts, pine nuts, and walnuts.

Limit dairy products and opt for yogurt, goat's milk, and goat cheese in moderation.

Favor white meat, poultry, and freshwater fish over beef, pork, and saltwater fish.

When to Buy Organic

I get asked all the time if it's necessary to buy organic. Organic foods, which are defined as being produced in soils free of synthetic chemicals, are now the fastest-growing sector of the food industry in much of the Western world. You can buy organic produce and organically grown grains, legumes, nuts, oils, sugars, wines, and a variety of other foods and beverages. Organic farming aims to avoid genetic modification, irradiation, and the use of sewer sludge as fertilizer. But is all of this worth the extra expense?

Here's my take on buying organic: I realize that for many people, buying everything organic is impractical, unrealistic, and expensive. It's also unnecessary. Some recent studies have even shown that organic foods do not impart any more nutrition than conventionally grown foods. That isn't to say that organic foods don't have other benefits, such as fewer synthetics and chemicals that can irritate your system. Not to mention the fact buying organic means you're likely supporting small farmers rather than large conglomerates. But it's worth noting that your diet and nutritional needs won't be "ruined" if you choose to buy only some organic foods. Also bear in mind that Ayurveda promotes eating fresh, vital food that's easy to digest. Whether or not you're choosing organic, the intrinsic nature of a certain food will either be light and easily digestible, such as produce and complex carbohydrates, or be naturally heavy and difficult to digest, such as red meat and other animal proteins. Even organic varieties of meats can lead to the formation of physical and mental toxins, or ama, due to the inherent chemical structure of meat. (It's well documented that direct correlations have been found between diets high in animal fat and illnesses such as obesity, heart disease, and cancer. This is true regardless of the "organic" label. When the body encounters hard-to-digest animal fat, especially the saturated kind, it converts it to fatty tissue and artery-clogging bad cholesterol.)

A general guideline to use is the following: Buy organic when you can, and especially when it comes to foods that you will eat with minimal processing or cooking and foods that are typically exposed to pesticides and herbicides when grown conventionally. Examples include fresh fruits and vegetables (especially those where you eat the skins), dairy, and grains. But don't discount the frozen food section; when you cannot afford fresh organic produce, chances are that frozen organic food will be less expensive. These foods are often picked at their peak of ripeness to preserve their nutrients; they are packed full of prana, the life force that bestows us energy and vitality.

So as much as possible, eat fresh, local, and seasonal, as this further attunes your body with the cycles of Mother Nature. Also be sure to avoid, as best you can, additives such as artificial sweeteners and colors, and ingredients you cannot pronounce or understand. In general, if the food comes with a nutrition label at all, it's been processed to some degree. The less packaging you have to get through to reach the food, the more natural your diet will be.

Timing Is Everything

Time your meals to maximize your body's inherent preferences for turning on its digestive fire. The ideal schedule:

- Breakfast between 7:00 and 8:00 a.m. Don't eat a lot of food after 9:00 a.m.
- Lunch (largest and most important meal of the day) between noon and 1:00 p.m.
- Dinner (which should consist of a light meal) before 7:00 p.m.
- Bedtime snack: If you need this, try a handful of berries or a piece of low-sugar fruit like an apple (not a banana).

Build and Maintain a Spice Rack

Perhaps there's no better way to liven up foods than to add a dash of spice or a pinch of fresh herbs. You don't have to run out and spend a fortune in one fell swoop to create a spice rack worthy of a cooking magazine cover, but here's a list of twenty-one items you'll want to start collecting and experimenting with in your dishes, in addition to the ones I've already mentioned that you'll use to prepare your basic khichadi and green tea blend (see page 102). Choose garden-fresh herbs and non-irradiated herbs and spices wherever possible. You can start just by purchasing an ounce of each of the herbs and spices you want to try; store them in their original containers or transfer them (especially if you buy them fresh without any packaging) to glass spice bottles that you can label.

1. Basil
2. Bay leaves
3. Black pepper
4. Broths (technically not a seasoning, but low-sodium chicken broth can add rich, tasty flavors to many dishes, including rice and vegetables)
5. Cayenne pepper (just a pinch added to meals has been shown to suppress appetite)
6. Chives
7. Cloves
8. Dill seeds
9. Fenugreek seeds
10. Mint
11. Mustard seeds, black and yellow
12. Oregano
13. Paprika
14. Parsley
15. Rosemary
16. Saffron
17. Sage
18. Sea salt
19. Tarragon
20. Thyme
21. Vanilla beans

To make the Hot Belly Diet easy to implement in your everyday eating life beyond the 30-day plan (see page 132) is a week-long menu plan with a multitude of original and highly versatile recipes. This menu plan will also help reinforce and demonstrate the recommendations provided in this chapter, as I show dishes that work well together and present a wide array of complementary side dishes, drinks, sauces, desserts, and condiments that incorporate a variety of the six tastes.

The number of meal ideas and recipes here goes to show how plentiful your choices are on this diet. You'll see an abundance of vegetables, fish, meat, poultry, nuts, eggs, and salads. But you could just as easily craft simpler dishes based on the themes presented here (e.g., pick a fish or meat to cook up with some side vegetables and a green salad for lunch or dinner and pack hard-boiled eggs for breakfast with a handful of nuts as a snack). You'll find a few ideas for dessert (yes, it's allowable!), as well as gourmet khichadi options when you have more time to play in the kitchen.

At www.hotbellydiet.com, you'll find my recommendations for specific brands of foods that follow the Hot Belly Diet guidelines. Even though you're evicting gluten, wheat, and most sugar from your diet, you'd be surprised by the abundance of food options available to you. You'll also be astonished by the control you'll gain over your hunger levels, cravings, portion sizes, and caloric intake. Your taste buds will be rejoicing, too, as they experience a rebirth of sorts and bestow upon you a new appreciation for food.

Notice that you won't find nutritional content information in these recipes. As I mentioned earlier, one of my goals in this book has been to liberate you from ever having to count calories or grams of protein and fat again. I want to teach you *how* to eat to keep your agni hot and healthy, not *what* to eat gram by gram and calorie by calorie. By now you should know the difference between a heavy, sticky meal and a light and energetic one. If you follow the guidelines and protocol, the fat, carbs, and protein intake will take care of itself. You won't overeat, you won't feel underfed, and you'll be maximally nourishing your body and soul.

In the past decade, there's been a huge shift in the variety of food available at our markets. If you live in an urban area, for instance, you're likely to be able to purchase any kind of ingredient within a matter of miles, whether that means visiting your usual grocery store that's now filled with organic foods or venturing to a local farmers' market. Get to know your grocers; they can tell you what just came in and where your foods are coming from. Aim for choosing produce that's in season, and be willing to try new foods you've never had before. Remember, go organic or wild whenever possible. When in doubt, ask your grocer.

Sample Menu for a Week
After the 30-Day Plan

Here is what a weeklong, Ayurvedic approach could look like. All dishes accompanied by recipes are in italics. The recipes begin on page 233. Note: You can use ghee, organic extra-virgin olive oil, sesame oil, or safflower oil when you panfry foods. Avoid processed oils and cooking sprays unless the spray is made from organic sources. Organic canola oil spray is fine for high-heat cooking. If you come across a dish that doesn't appeal to you, simply choose another like-minded one. Appendix A is filled with extra recipes to suit different tastes and preferences.

Monday

➤ Breakfast: Sprouted wheat bread with almond butter + 2 eggs scrambled with 1 cup cleansing vegetables (see page 98) and leafy greens
➤ Lunch: *Persimmon Salad with Fennel* with 3 to 4 ounces of lean protein + *Mint Tea*
➤ Dinner: *Pumpkin Soup* + *Tossed Arugula Salad*
➤ Dessert: Whole grain chocolate chip cookies and a cup of chamomile tea

Tuesday

➤ Breakfast: *Hot Quinoa Cereal with Warm Spiced Milk*
➤ Lunch: Whole grain pasta with stir-fried vegetables and *Cilantro Pesto Sauce* + *Kale and Cranberry Salad*
➤ Dinner: Baked fish with ½ cup brown or basmati rice and steamed vegetables
➤ Dessert: 1 serving dark chocolate

Wednesday

➤ Breakfast: *Superfood Smoothie* + 1 hard-boiled egg (optional)
➤ Lunch: 3 to 4 ounces grilled sirloin steak with *Lemon-Roasted Asparagus* + ½ cup cooked wild or basmati rice
➤ Dinner: Soup and salad of your choice
➤ Dessert: 1 serving of *Stewed Apples with Cloves and Cinnamon*

Thursday

➤ Breakfast: Veggie scramble with 2 whole eggs, 1 egg white, and 2 cleansing vegetables (see page 98)
➤ Lunch: *Black Bean Tacos with Mango Salsa*

➤ Dinner: *Suppertime Khichadi* + *Citrusy Kale Salad with Blueberries and Pumpkin Seeds*
➤ Dessert: (Skipped!)

Friday

➤ Breakfast: *Yogurt Parfait with Low-Fat Granola*
➤ Lunch: *Butternut Squash and Spinach Curry* + 3 ounces of lean protein
➤ Dinner: *Asparagus Soup* + salad of choice
➤ Dessert: Small bowl of fresh fruit

Saturday

➤ Breakfast: *Coconut-Cucumber Smoothie* + 1 hard-boiled egg
➤ Lunch: *Braised Chicken with Cilantro-Reduction Sauce* + ½ cup wild rice + steamed veggies
➤ Dinner: *Kale and Mandarin Salad* + soup of choice
➤ Dessert: 1 serving tapioca pudding

Sunday

➤ Breakfast: Bowl of steel-cut oatmeal topped with fresh berries
➤ Lunch: 3 ounces of lean protein + 1 cup of steamed cleansing vegetables (see page 98) + ½ cup cooked quinoa or brown rice
➤ Dinner: *Gourmet Khichadi*
➤ Dessert: 2 scoops of sorbet

Eating Anywhere

As you segue into the second month, work toward the goal of being able to eat anywhere and not always have your own food on hand. You can do this even if you haven't reached your ideal weight yet. Most of us find ourselves eating outside our homes a lot, especially while we're at work. It's virtually impossible to plan and prepare every single meal, so strive to navigate other menus with confidence and resolve. Aim to enjoy your favorite restaurants and order off the menu while still following my guidelines. If it's too challenging, then explore new restaurants. It's actually not that hard to make any menu work for you once you get used to certain substitutions and seeking foods that match the guiding principles. Broiled chicken or fish with steamed vegetables and brown rice is likely to be a safe bet (skip the fried foods, heavy gravies and dressings, and ask for a starter salad with olive oil and vinegar or a cup of brothy soup). Beware of elaborate dishes that contain a long list of ingredients and heavy sauces. Whenever you're in doubt about a particular menu item, either skip it or ask your server about it.

In general, minimize how many times you eat out because eliminating all sources of unhealthy, ama-producing ingredients is impossible. On most days of the week, commit to consuming foods that you prepare. Once you've gotten a handle on this way of eating, see if you can go back to your old recipes and modify them to fit my guidelines. You'd be surprised by what a little experimentation in the kitchen can do to turn a classic dish filled with heavy, ama-building ingredients into an equally delicious but agni-friendly meal. Instead of processed (refined) wheat flours, try flours made from coconut, nut meals like ground almonds, and ground flaxseed; in lieu of white sugar, find ways to sweeten your recipes with Stevia, honey, or whole fruits; and rather than cooking with processed oils, stick with ghee and extra-virgin olive oil.

Keeping the Fires Burning Brightly

As with so many things in life, maintaining a newly established habit takes commitment and effort. It's a balancing act to keep good habits dominating even when old habits try to reemerge. Once you've shifted your dietary protocol and changed the way you buy, cook, and order food, you'll still have moments when you'll give in to temptations. I don't expect you to never eat processed food, fast food, or a steak dinner again, but I do hope that you stay mindful of your body's true needs, now that you have the knowledge, and live out this newly found sensibility every day as best you can. We all know that splurges are bound to happen, so don't beat yourself up when you're faced with temptation (e.g., the pizza and box of pastries at work or a friend's birthday cake). But do remind yourself that they are indeed splurges and accept any potential consequences if you cannot say no.

Although many people try to eat well 80 percent of the time and leave the last 20 percent for splurges, I find that all too often people are doing the opposite—eating poorly for the majority of the time. This happens, quite frankly, automatically and inadvertently as we let the occasional splurge morph into a regular habit, and we find ourselves faced with endless excuses such as parties, weddings, a stressful day at work or just Friday night. There will always be an available (and reasonably-sounding) excuse for not taking better care of yourself. This is life, and accepting a little give-and-take is okay. So aim to stick to a 90/10 rule. For 90 percent of the time, eat within my guidelines and let the last 10 percent take care of itself. And whenever you feel like your body needs another reboot, you can just return to the main protocol of the Hot Belly Diet for a month. This simple plan can always be your lifeline to a healthier way of living that supports the vision you have for yourself—and your body.

Life is a treasure trove of decisions, some of which are harder to make than others. *Right or left? Today or tomorrow? Yes or no?* Hopefully the good decisions trump the bad ones. My ultimate goal in writing this book is to show you how to make better choices that will allow you to fully participate in life. My hope is that I've given you plenty of ideas to at least begin to make a positive difference in your body's innate healing powers. Every day in my practice I witness the value that being healthy brings to people. I also see what sudden illness and chronic disease can do, regardless of their achievements and how much they are loved. Put simply, when you're vibrantly healthy, possibilities abound.

PART TWO

Light

CHAPTER 7

The Ancient Exercise to Create a Fat-Burning, Fit Body Without Strain

Exercise is one of the most powerful tools to slow down aging.

—CHARAKA

I f you could go back in time to see how ancient cultures sat down, you'd notice that many sat upright on floors in the cross-legged position, kneeled, or sat with "tent knees" as do many Africans today, with their buttocks and feet on the ground, knees bent. These positions require a level of strength in the legs, glutes, and back, as well as balance and coordination. Only in relatively recent times have we employed the use of chairs and couches that have the unfortunate effect of putting the body in positions that lead to pelvic stagnation and reduced circulatory function. The way we sit today is not ideal for our body's natural mechanics, and it's no wonder that we are increasingly finding ourselves diagnosed with "sitting diseases" ranging from nagging lower back pain to serious conditions such as diabetes and even heart disease. The connection between sitting in a seat for most of the day and developing serious maladies isn't that difficult to make, in fact. Think about it: Most of us spend more than eight hours a day at a desk job, at least one hour a day commuting, and several hours more either sleeping or engaged in a primarily sedentary activity such as eating, watching television, or just milling about. The science of this relationship is actually quite new, and it's astonishing; we'll be exploring it shortly.

So let's do a little experiment: Without worrying about how fast you're moving, can you sit on the floor and then rise up to a standing position using as little support as possible? Turns out that if you can get yourself up from the floor using just one hand—or even better, without the help of any hand—then you're not only in the higher percentile of musculoskeletal fitness, but you're much more likely to live longer than those who can't do this exercise. In 2012 a study performed in Brazil at an exercise medicine clinic and published in the *European Journal of Preventive Cardiology* (formerly called the *European Journal of Cardiovascular Prevention and Rehabilitation*) revealed that the ability to sit and get up from the floor is closely related to all-cause mortality risk (another way of saying "dying from anything"). Put simply, the better you can do this task without relying on your hands for stability and support, the longer you'll live. The findings are hardly inconsequential. It is well known that aerobic fitness is strongly associated with survival, but this study also shows that maintaining high levels of flexibility, muscular strength, and coordination have a positive influence on life expectancy (not to mention that they make daily activities easier to do). Being able to stand up from the floor without extra support requires a strong lower body, including strong ankles, knees, and calves. It also demands that our lower body from our hips down be open and flexible. And today's lifestyles have many of us going in the other direction—toward crippling stagnation.

When people ask me for the "one piece of advice" that's good for all three doshas, or body types, regardless of age or the season, I like to refer to the legendary story of when Charaka, the father of Ayurveda, was asked the same question by a boy thousands of years ago. His response: "Wake up in the morning and go for a walk at sunrise." Today we know the power of such an activity on the body's health and longevity. Although now we use high-tech words like "neuroplasticity" to describe how the brain positively responds to physical movement (and how, for instance, the simple act of walking, which spurs the birth of new brain cells, allows you to literally walk your way to a new brain), the modern science has been known by ancient lore for a long, long time. It's just that today we have fancy tools and methods for proving what the ancients already knew. And while we may act surprised when we read a headline that says we're more likely to crave sugary and salty foods when we're sedentary, which, of course, is linked to weight gain and heart trouble, this logic has also been known since the sages of yesteryear first wrote about the value of physical exercise on health. From an Ayurvedic point of view, exercise can be seen as even more important than food. Indeed, food provides prana, or energy. But if your body's energy channels are clogged and blocked, if your system is congested and the flow of blood, hormones, and other substances is not ideal, then you cannot use that food efficiently and absorb all its nutrients. Exercise facilitates the intelligent communication between cells, pure and simple.

I know that I'm not the first to tell you that exercise is an antidote for nearly every ailment. It improves everything about us from our digestion and metabolism to our appearance, body tone and strength, and bone density. It also helps us normalize weight and feel good about ourselves. It can literally turn on our "smart genes," de-age us, support emotional stability and stave off depression, and help make healthier eating choices all the easier. But I want to be the first to share with you some starling new research on the science of exercise that fits within the model of an Ayurvedic approach to life. I also want to give you the motivation and instructions you need to make a regular exercise routine happily doable, because fewer than 20 percent of the population make this a habit. Although we have a tendency in the West to think of all exercise as good exercise,

Ayurveda encourages a slightly different perspective. Your particular body type, age, strength, and physical condition are among the factors you should consider in choosing activities that get your heart rate up and blood flowing faster. I'll be giving you a program in this chapter that works for everyone, but I trust that this can serve as a strong foundation for customizing your particular routine in the future. The goal is to find a personal fitness routine that brings balance to your mind and body, that respects your physical limitations, and that doesn't cause undue strain, harm, or overexertion.

As much as we see an abundance of anti-exercisers today, we also see a lot of people becoming fanatical about their exercise. Extreme sports and athletic competitions have gained enormous popularity in the last decade. But those who become exercise radicals likely have an underlying doshic imbalance, as well as psychological and emotional issues. High-pitta types, for instance, can push themselves to the point of injury. High-vata types are often attracted to exercises that entail constant, fast movement and changing stimuli. High-kapha types may not want to exercise at all, even though they are the ideal body type for more vigorous, challenging forms of exercise. While it's common for us to turn to demanding exercise in pursuit of the perfect body or to release our pent-up emotions, in my world, that's when it's best to turn inward through practices such as yoga and deep breathing.

In this chapter, first we're going to take a tour of exercise's positive forces on the body from a very modern, scientific perspective. Then we'll circle back to how the latest science corroborates what Ayurveda has been teaching for centuries, and I'll guide you toward finding a routine that works with your schedule and preferences. I'll also give some dosha-specific tips for those of you who are interested in matching activities with your individual constitution. It goes without saying that physical movement is a cornerstone to an Ayurvedic way of life. Just as a fiery flow of agni is key to health, so is constant physical movement in your life. If you can imagine there

The Magic of Movement

The following benefits of exercise have long been proven scientifically. There's ample proof that working the body physically lights up the energy powers from within and has benefits that go far beyond the mere physical:

- Increased stamina, strength, and flexibility
- Increased coordination
- Increased blood circulation and oxygen supply to cells and tissues
- More restful, sound sleep
- Balanced hormones
- Stress reduction, mood stability, lower incidence of depression
- Higher self-esteem and sense of well-being
- Increased muscle tone and bone health
- Release of brain chemicals called endorphins that act as natural mood lifters and pain relievers
- Decreased food cravings
- Decreased blood sugar levels and risk for diabetes
- Ideal weight distribution and maintenance
- Increased brain health, sharper memory, lower risk for dementia
- Increased heart health, lower risk for cardiovascular disease
- Decreased inflammation and risk for age-related disease, including cancer
- Increased energy and productivity
- Increased longevity and happiness

being a warm fire burning bright in your belly, then you can understand why it's important to have a vent of air coming in to keep that fire burning. And that vent is possible through exercise, which, of course, promotes a fiery, robust circulation to constantly rekindle that fire. But don't panic: I won't ask you to start running marathons or even join a gym. I will lay out a simple program that you can do from the comfort of your home and that won't be overly aggressive, time-sucking, or exhausting. This will include a combination of a basic yoga practice and a cardio routine. Before we even get to those details, though, let me make my case for commencing an exercise program, however minimal or ambitious you'd like it to be.

How the "Skinny-Fat Syndrome" Sounded the Alarm in the Twenty-First Century

Throughout most of human history, we've been physically active during the day in both our personal and professional lives. But as I've already hinted at, today modern technology has afforded us the privilege of a sedentary existence; virtually anything we need is available at our fingertips and our jobs have many of us sedentary at a desk. Science has even proven that our genome, over millions of years, evolved in a state of constant physical challenge—it took effort to find food just to survive. So our genome expects and requires frequent exercise. Some of the latest science has actually revealed that we are designed to be active so that we can live long enough to procreate. Evolutionary biologists now purport that we've survived this long on earth as a result of our athletic prowess. When our cavemen ancestors outran predators and hunted down valuable prey for food, this essentially facilitated our continual existence on the planet. We were able to procure meals and energy for mating, which could then allow those early active humans to pass on their genes to the next generation of stronger, hardier humans.

But, unfortunately, too few of us meet the physical demands our body expects today, and our high rates of chronic illness are evidence. Contrary to popular wisdom, diabetes and high cholesterol are not just problems attributable to overweight and obese individuals. Take thirty-year-old Shelly as an example. Her story mirrors those of so many others I've treated. She had a body most women idolized, and never had to work hard to maintain her figure at 5'8" and 130 pounds. She dined on lots of salads and saved light exercise for the weekends. Prior to coming to see me, she'd been hit with debilitating fatigue that her primary care doctor had originally thought was a thyroid problem. But tests revealed that there was nothing wrong with her thyroid. The problem was found in her blood sugar levels, which indicated she was prediabetic.

Shelly was shocked. She knew diabetes was a health crisis, but didn't think she'd be among the statistics. According to the Centers for Disease Control and Prevention, nearly twenty-six million Americans have the disease, including millions of people who don't know it and have yet to be diagnosed. Shelly couldn't understand how she could be on the verge of type 2 diabetes since she wasn't outwardly fat and didn't have a junky diet. What was the culprit? Put another way, what was her missing ingredient to health?

The CDC estimates that the numbers are just going to get worse. Although one in nine adults has diabetes today, we're trending toward one in three by the year 2050. For decades, we envisioned typical type 2 patients as being what Shelly imagined: overweight (or obese) with an allergy to exercise. We also pictured people who are older, often receiving a diagnosis in middle age or beyond. No doubt these type 2 cases among older, overweight folks continue to climb, but there has been a disturbing increase in a much younger, "thinner" set.

In the past ten years, the number of hospitalizations among people in their thirties who have diabetes-related problems has doubled. What's more troubling is the epic number of people aged twenty or older with prediabetes: sixty-five million, up from fifty-seven million in 2007. So a serious condition that used to take half a lifetime to develop is now afflicting young people. Perhaps even more astonishing is the fact that roughly 15 percent of type 2 diabetics are of normal weight. They look healthy on the outside but are hiding a dark secret that could be unbeknownst to them.

Shelly's story is symbolic of a growing problem that I see every day—thin on the outside, fat on the inside. And her medical condition can mostly be blamed on one thing: lack of physical movement. Not only is her body's stagnation negatively affecting her biochemistry, but she's missing out on many of the wondrous positive effects that movement can have on her ability to process food and maintain a healthy-energy metabolism. In fact, an alarming increase in the number of cases like Shelly is cluing us in to just how important it is to exercise *regardless of weight*. These cases may at first seem like outliers, but they are sounding the alarm on the hazards of shunning exercise, as well as the benefits of movement.

So what's going on beneath the surface of someone like Shelly? How can her looks defy the dysfunction stewing within? This condition, which can be virtually impossible to detect from a person's outer appearance, develops when fat that would normally accumulate under your skin sticks to your abdominal organs instead. This visceral fat is much worse than any upper-arm flab or "thunder thighs"; it can instigate inflammatory substances that adversely affect your liver and pancreas, and lower your insulin sensitivity. As a result, you become increasingly vulnerable to type 2 diabetes. Indeed, looks can be deceiving: You might look svelte on the outside, but if we were to peek inside at your physiology, we'd find an environment typically seen in the obese.

As it turns out, shunning exercise and controlling weight through food choices alone is the likely culprit here. In order to shrink visceral fat and lower blood sugar, physical movement is essential. And the science now proves that even moderate exercise can foster rapid consumption of blood sugar by muscles (i.e., they will consume glucose at twenty times their normal rate). According to the National Institutes of Health (NIH), and based on studies, just thirty minutes of brisk walking a day can slash your odds of developing type 2 diabetes by more than 50 percent. This is true even for people who are already prediabetic. Another big culprit is yo-yo dieting. When you lose weight quickly through calorie restriction, you don't just lose fat. You also lose muscle. And when you regain that weight, most of that gain is in the form of fat. So there's an overall loss of precious muscle—muscle that would help one to burn visceral fat and control blood sugar. This scenario is a set up for type 2 diabetes.

In addition to these risks is the impact of daily stress. Too much stress will trigger your body to produce more of the stress hormone cortisol. But cortisol won't just help to energize you; it will temporarily elevate your blood sugar. Hence, if you're tense all the time, you're in the danger zone for diabetes. What's more, we know that too much cortisol can also interfere with fat storage, which is why people who are of normal weight but are stressed out all the time can actually have higher amounts of invisible visceral fat. Indeed, chronic stress can make you skinny-fat.

And just what exactly is visceral fat? I've used the term a few times without proper definition.

Bad Belly Bulge

We used to think that fat cells were just biological garages for storing excess calories that could be tapped for energy when needed. But we know better now. Fat cells do much more than simply sit on the sidelines holding quiet calories. They form masses of complex, sophisticated hormonal organs that are very much involved in human physiology and that can be considered organs themselves.

Your body's collective fat mass could very well be one of your most industrious organs, serving a lot of functions far beyond keeping you insulated and cushioned. This is especially true of that so-called visceral fat that surrounds your abdominal "visceral" organs such as the kidneys, pancreas, heart, liver, and intestines. You've probably heard of visceral fat since it has made many headlines in the media over the past few years. Although we may wish to get rid of cellulite and the fat on our thunder thighs, upper arms, and buttocks, the kind of fat that we doctors worry about the most is that which hugs the internal organs and may not be visible from the outside. (Though in overweight and obese individuals, paunches and thick waistlines are the outward signs of high visceral fat levels.)

Contrary to the fat that shapes our butts and thighs, visceral fat is like a live wire. It's very metabolically active, releasing fatty acids, inflammatory agents, and hormones that ultimately lead to elevated bad cholesterol, triglycerides, blood glucose, and blood pressure. It's what makes obesity so harmful, because unlike the fat just under our skin (subcutaneous fat), visceral fat unleashes its metabolic products such as excess triglycerides directly into the bloodstream, carrying them to the liver where they get dumped as free fatty acids. Free fatty acids also collect in the pancreas, heart, and other vital organs—places that are not meant to store fat. The result is organ dysfunction, which handicaps the healthy control of insulin, blood sugar, and cholesterol levels. And all of this activity triggers inflammatory pathways. Adding insult to injury, studies now show that visceral fat not only generates inflammation through a chain of biological events, but also becomes inflamed itself.

(For the record, although obesity has only recently been declared a "disease" by the medical community in the U.S., it's been recognized as a serious malady for centuries among medical practitioners. In fact, prehistoric Indian scriptures point to a lack of physical activity as the number one cause of obesity, followed by daytime sleep, excess fat intake, and excess alcohol consumption. All of these causes are further tied to metabolic challenges that don't allow the proper utilization of fat in the body. In Ayurveda, obesity is called *medo roga*, and more broadly speaking, Ayurveda holds agni responsible for obesity: When agni is impaired, then the ama, or toxic substances, is built up in the body, leading to obesity. Obese kings in ancient India would be sent away to work in the fields to reverse their condition. Obesity may be called a modern scourge due to its prevalence, but it has plagued millions of humans for millennia. Only now are we also beginning to see how the ravages of obesity can be detected in seemingly "healthy" individuals.)

Thankfully, Shelly managed to experience a medical transformation in her health without resorting to drugs. She started to make exercise a regular routine throughout the week and reduced her consumption of white flour and processed sugars. She watched her blood sugar levels drop to nearly normal, an indication that she was making headway at burning off damaging, visceral fat, and getting her inflammatory pathways under control.

If cautionary tales like Shelly's aren't enough to motivate you about the magic of movement, then let me take you closer to the science of exercise that proves why we must move, and move often. But we don't have to be nearly as ambitious as someone who plans to compete in an athletic event. It turns out that a little can go a long way, so long as we're not sitting for prolonged periods of time.

Walk Your Body to Jog Your Genes and Run Your Mind

Exercise physiology has come a long way in the last twenty years. We know so much more about the mechanics of the human body through laboratory and clinical tests that show us exactly what's going on when we move to the point of panting and sweating. Entire new fields of medicine have emerged, such as metabolomics, which is a form of metabolic profiling that aims to find patterns in people that either spell disease or lower their risk for certain illnesses. Out of this new field has come the compelling finding that the more physically fit you are, the more benefits you reap in terms of your metabolism. One case in point: In a 2010 study, Boston researchers from Massachusetts General Hospital and the Broad Institute (of MIT and Harvard) found that fit people, as opposed to unfit people, have greater increases in certain metabolites in their bodies that affect how calories and fat get burned and how cells respond to stress, as well as how blood sugar is controlled. It turns out that the very act of exercise itself can change our internal chemistry down to biomolecules that factor heavily into whether we have a healthy and fast or, conversely, unhealthy and sluggish metabolism.

One of the most captivating areas of study taking place today is how exercise can change the expression of your genes and literally reverse the aging process. That's right: Exercise can change how your DNA "acts." DNA may be static, but how your DNA speaks to your body through its encoded genes is anything but fixed. Like switches, genes can turn on or off in response to cues coming from elsewhere in the body and delivered via biochemical signals. Genes in the "on" mode express various proteins that trigger a specific range of physiological actions in the body; likewise, genes in the "off" mode usually prevent certain reactions from happening, which can be a good thing or not.

In 2008 a group of Canadian and American researchers studied the effects of strength training for six months in people aged sixty-five and older. They took small biopsies of muscle cells from the seniors' thighs before and after the six-month period, and compared them with muscle cells from twenty-six individuals whose average age was twenty-two. The scientists documented evidence that the program improved the seniors' strength by 50 percent, which was to be expected. But they also documented significant changes at the genetic level. At the beginning of the six-month period, the researchers had recorded discrepancies in the expression of six hundred genes between the older and younger participants. This means that these genes are associated with age, becoming more or less active over time. By the end of the exercise period, though, the expression of a third of those genes had changed. Put simply, the genetic profile of the sexagenarians who'd gone through the strength-training program resembled that of the twentysomething group. Upon closer inspection, the researchers figured out that the genes that changed were involved in the functioning of mitochondria, which are your body's most important energy packagers. These little structures, which contain their own DNA, are found inside every cell and are responsible for converting the energy in food into ATP—the molecule that provides chemical energy for physiological processes.

The health of your mitochondria is paramount to your general health, for their age and ability to perform have a direct correlation with your metabolic health. And they are also exceptionally vulnerable to cellular damage, which can result from a number of things both under your control and not. In addition to your eating habits and environmental exposures affecting your mitochondria's functionality and health, the amount of exercise you get also plays a vital role. Studies show that aerobic exercise for just fifteen to twenty minutes at a moderate intensity, done just three to four times a week, can increase the number of mitochondria in your muscle cells by a whopping 40 to 50 percent. That's quite an exchange: a little bit of exercise for a huge increase in the amount of these little engines that rev up your energy metabolism and help to burn fat.

A conversation about the positive genetic changes that can occur with exercise wouldn't be complete without bringing up how physical activity can also impact the brain. And again we can turn to new science to prove this point. For a long time, we've known that exercise is good for the brain, but only in the past decade have we really been able to quantify and qualify the extraordinary relationship between physical and mental fitness. It's been scientifically demonstrated that aerobic exercise in particular not only turns on genes linked to longevity, but also causes your brain to turn up production of certain brain chemicals known to have positive health effects, including those that stave off depression and enhance processing power. What's more, it targets a specific gene that's related to the brain's internal "growth hormone." Aerobic exercise has also been shown to reverse memory decline in elderly humans, and actually increase growth of new brain cells in the brain's memory center (gives a whole new meaning to the phrase "jog your memory"). Eons ago, we thrived across the planet because we could outpace predators and other animals vying for precious resources. This ultimately helped make us the clever, big-brained human beings we are today. The more we moved, the smarter we got. Which is probably another reason why being sedentary, or just chronically desk-bound, can be so damaging to health.

Sickened by Sitting

While I was writing this book, the headlines reported that sitting was the new smoking. I had to laugh at this provocative analogy because I felt like I'd known this for a long time. Old wisdom passed down for generations in my culture says that no matter how fit you are, if you sit for most of the day, you are likely going to experience poor health and meet an early death. But now we have modern science to validate the evidence that's been anecdotally known forever.

The public seemed awed by this news, but perhaps it's difficult to see how even an hour daily spent working out rigorously won't erase the effects of sitting down for most of the remainder of the day. But a growing body of emerging research is revealing that it's entirely possible to get plenty of physical activity and still suffer significant increases in your risk of death and disease—just like smoking harms no matter how much you engage in other, healthier lifestyle habits.

Exercising won't erase the negative effects of smoking, and neither will sitting on your derriere for prolonged periods, which so many of us do today as we barely move an inch to go from home, car, work, and back again to sit on the couch and watch TV.

The reason sitting is such a health offender when performed in large doses is due to the biological effects that take place in the body as a result. Sitting for extended periods, *independent of physical activity,* has been shown to have significant metabolic consequences, negatively influencing resting blood pressure and healthy levels of triglycerides (blood fats), high-density lipoprotein (the "good" cholesterol), blood sugar, and the appetite hormone leptin, all of which are factors in obesity and other chronic diseases. Leptin is one of the body's metabolic hormones. Among its many actions, it tells you when to pull away from the table and stop eating.

The studies confirming the connection between sitting time and total mortality began to emerge in the last decade. One of the first alarming studies came from researchers at the American Cancer Society who published a paper in the *American Journal of Epidemiology* that equated sitting with smoking or overexposure to the sun. Women who said they sat for more than six hours per day were 37 percent more likely to die during the time period studied than those who sat fewer than three hours a day. Men who were on their butts more than six hours a day were 18 percent more likely to die from heart disease and had a 7.8 percent increased chance of dying from diabetes compared with someone who sat for three hours or less a day. And these were all hours tabulated outside of work. Even when the researchers adjusted for physical activity level, the association remained virtually unchanged. Another study that soon followed at the Baker IDI Heart and Diabetes Institute in Melbourne concluded that even two hours of exercise a day would not make up for sitting most of the day.

And that was just the beginning. We can turn to many studies today that uphold the same conclusion: Sitting supports sickness.

In 2013 yet another study revealed that people who walked for four hours daily and stood for two had greater insulin sensitivity—a good thing for reducing risk for diabetes and heart disease—than those who completed an intense workout for an hour but who were otherwise sedentary. What explains this? The forces placed on the body during sustained movement trigger the release of enzymes that help regulate blood-sugar balance.

The biological reasoning behind the sitting-sickness connection makes total sense from another perspective, too: When you're sedentary, blood circulation slows. This means you're utilizing less blood sugar and burning less fat, and it turns out that you're also affecting your genes. Marc Hamilton, PhD, professor and director of the Inactivity Physiology Department at Pennington Biomedical Research Center in Baton Rouge, Louisiana, has found that an important gene called "lipid phosphate phosphatase-1," or "LPP1," which aids in the health of your cardiovascular system, is quite literally turned off when you sit for a few hours. And exercise won't necessarily turn this gene on if your muscles have been idle most of the day. In other words, LPP1 won't be influenced by exercise, but it will be changed by sitting, resulting in adverse outcomes. Dr. Hamilton has also reported that regardless of whether or not people exercised the recommended 150 minutes a week, they still spent an average of sixty-four hours a week sitting, twenty-eight hours standing, and eleven hours walking in a manner that could not remotely qualify as exercise.

In a study spanning twelve years on more than seventeen thousand Canadians, scientists discovered that the more time people spent sitting, the younger they died despite their body weight or how much they exercised.

What these latest studies are showing is that prolonged sitting isn't just a risk factor for diabetes and heart disease. It's tied to an increased risk for depression and cancer, too. And again, the physiological reasoning makes sense: When you're relatively motionless, your circulation is reduced, and so is the flow of certain substances in the blood that keep us feeling good and that police inflammatory pathways. Feel-good hormones that are linked to our mood and keep us happy and optimistic cannot bathe the brain, which is partly why it's long been known that one way to change your attitude is to just get off your butt and get a good dose of physical activity. Or just go for a walk around the block!

What to Do: Move, Breathe, Sweat, Repeat

Now that I've given you a crash course in the latest exercise physiology, let's bring this discussion back to the concept of Ayurveda as I explain just how to put these ideas and facts of inspiration to good use.

Ayurevda's approach to exercise can best be summed up by turning to Charaka, the greatest writer on Ayurveda, who once said that from physical exercise we get lightness, a capacity for work, tolerance of difficulties, elimination of impurities, and stimulation of digestion. Engaging in cardio (aerobics) and resistance training (use of weights) can help you to achieve some of these goals, but they won't be enough to satisfy Charaka's description. Ideally, we want to balance the whole system, which includes both the mind and the body. It's also key that exercise gives more than it takes. In other words, it should infuse you with energy, not rob you of it and leave you depleted. After all, life is meant to be comfortable and pleasant, and as such, Ayurveda respects exercise as a means to that end. While some people view exercise as work, Ayurveda sees it as a primer for work. It should render you livelier, more alert, and clearheaded—ready for work! The commonly touted mantra of "no pain, no gain" is just a myth.

Of all the options available today for exercise, I have to admit that walking still reigns supreme. It's among the most natural of activities and caters to all three doshas. Pitta types love the sensation of being slowed down, since they spend much of their day working at a fast pace. Vata types feel tranquilized by it. And kapha types are often stimulated by walking, feeling lighter and less congested. Because walking uses both sides of the body (you're using both the left and right in balance), it dovetails all the pairing that Ayurveda honors. From an Ayurvedic standpoint, everything in life is paired. Not only do we have right and left, but we have hot and cold, the sun and moon, the masculine and feminine, the sympathetic and parasympathetic nervous system, stimulating substances and calming ones, a pair of eyes and ears, and let's not forget the yin and yang. In fact, such natural pairings in nature is partly why yoga is so revered; it entails a combination of poses that work one side, then the other. The essence of Ayurveda is about regulating opposites—opening up opposing channels and balancing everything out. And plain old walking serves a mighty role in this regard, too. Walking has so many healing properties that I recommend it to my patients as a starter exercise if they haven't been active in a while. I also advise that a twenty-minute walk become a routine after every meal, a prescription I've already given in Part 1.

If there's one thing that separates an Ayurvedic approach to exercise from the more modern perspective is that exercise needn't put strain on the body or make you feel like you're forcing the body to do something it doesn't want to do. This isn't about pounding your muscles into shape. Exercise is not a "necessary evil" in the name of health. Much to the contrary, exercise aims to bring you closer to yourself—your physical body as well as your ethereal sense of self. It should be energizing, invigorating, enlivening, and eternally calming. And there's no better way to achieve these things than to incorporate three important activities into your life. I've already mentioned one of them, walking. This is a form of cardio to get your heart rate up (we like to say that cardio makes your heart muscles dance with joy). The other two are yoga and deep breathing.

So to this end, let me outline my suggested protocol for you, which you can begin on Day 1 of the program. Note that highly strenuous workouts are strongly discouraged in Phase 1 and 2 while you are purging and resetting your body. You can incorporate heavy weight training, any rigorous gym routine, or high cardio back into your life starting in Phase 3 and beyond.

Walking: As recommended in the program, aim to walk for at least twenty minutes after each meal, within minutes of finishing your last bite. This will stimulate your body's flow of healthy biomolecules, and, of course, the agni. As a general rule, you want to walk at a brisk pace that compels your heart and lungs to work harder than usual. You're not exerting yourself to the point where you're sweating heavily and panting for breath, but you're breaking a light sweat and starting to breathe through your mouth. In light of the 30-day theme, here's how to make the most of thirty minutes:

> First ten minutes: Walk at a moderate, warm-up pace
> Next ten minutes: Take up the tempo and walk at a brisk pace
> Final ten minutes: Maintain a moderate pace

Additional Cardio: If you've led a primarily sedentary life until commencing the Hot Belly Diet, then by all means it's perfectly fine to stick with a simple walking routine until you feel comfortable experimenting with other types of exercises that get your heart rate up. But if you want an added challenge or you're a seasoned exerciser, then I recommend incorporating other forms of moderate cardio work into your week. Aim for at least thirty minutes of formal cardio three times weekly (which can be in addition to your semi-leisurely walks after your meals). Your cardio routines can entail any number of activities, from the use of a machine such as an elliptical or stationary bike to actually going out for a bike ride, swimming laps, or taking an aerobics class. The goal is to exercise up to 50 percent of your maximum capacity (e.g., if you know that you can jog four miles, make it two miles; if you can swim twenty laps, make it ten laps). Again, make it a goal to work your cardiovascular system harder than usual, but not to the point where you're panting through your mouth and would have a hard time simultaneously talking to someone else while exercising. This guideline will keep you from crossing the threshold above which you're overly exerting your body and making exercise less efficient. This also keeps you in the ideal zone for maximizing the Hot Belly Diet's results. If you overdo your exercise, you'll burn out quickly and might not make it to the finish line. (Warning: Vata types can easily overdo their workouts because they naturally have lower exercise thresholds than pitta types, and pittas have lower thresholds than kaphas. Respect your dosha. Consider your age as well: If you're over the age of forty-five or fifty, be extra careful about overexerting yourself. Everyone begins to have increased vata starting in middle age, so one needs to balance out this dosha or you will experience an aggravated vata that can invite health challenges.)

The best time of day to engage in your cardio is either early in the morning or early in the evening (i.e., dawn or dusk). These are transitional periods for the day. In the morning, you're shedding the heaviness of the night, and activity will stimulate you for the day. In the evening, you're rejuvenating your body after the long day while at the same time preparing it for restful sleep. We have an old saying in the Vedic language that translates to "the quality of rest decides the quality of activity and vice versa."

Yoga: By Phase 2, aim to start a basic yoga practice two or three times a week (e.g., every three days). I realize that for some of you, this may sound like a huge effort if you've never tried yoga before, but you can simply start at home in front of your television or com-

Dosha-Specific Activities

Vata: Go for exercises that are gentle and flowing in nature, such as low-impact aerobics, bicycling, swimming, dancing, and tai chi.

Pitta: So long as pitta types don't overdo it or become extremely competitive in athletic competitions (e.g., marathons, triathlons), they do well with most forms of exercise, including bicycling, surfing, skiing, playing soccer, tennis, basketball, and engaging in martial arts and weight-lifting.

Kapha: Aim for stimulating exercises that harness your strength and endurance, such as aerobics, bicycling, jogging/running, rock climbing, rowing, and playing tennis or basketball.

puter using a video (for ideas, go to www.hotbellydiet.com). Yoga has become so mainstream today that you'd be hard-pressed to live in a place that doesn't offer at least one type of yoga class; it has become one of the most popular forms of exercise in the West.

In Sanskrit, *yoga* means "union" or "yoke" and refers to the union of mind and body. Broadly speaking, it also relates to one's union with the higher self or the Divine. Although yoga is typically known in Western culture as a practice that highlights physical postures and breathing techniques, it's a complete system of spiritual development that's designed to simultaneously work and purify the body while promoting self-discovery.

Start with a Level 1 class that introduces you to the main poses, then you can graduate to more advanced classes and see which type of yoga you like best. Classic Ashtanga and Vinyasa (or "flow yoga") classes are probably the most popular today (and versions thereof, such as "power yoga" and "hot yoga," which is a class in a high-temp room). But if you're a beginner, just start by choosing a class that offers the fundamentals.

The experience of yoga reinforces the goals of the Hot Belly Diet:

- ➤ To encourage a sense of lightness and clarity.
- ➤ To burn fat and build healthy tissues, including muscles.
- ➤ To improve connections among the various systems of the body, including its core hormonal functions that affect everything about us, from our cues of hunger and fullness to those that direct our immune system and cellular repair.
- ➤ To release unwanted toxins in tissues, and delete unwanted, depressive thoughts through yoga's mindfulness. It's no wonder that science can now prove how anger impairs the liver, fear triggers the kidneys, and a lack of love weakens the heart.
- ➤ To get rid of excess fluids and water that are dampening the cellular fires of the body and slowing down metabolic activity, as the movements of yoga help address edema in the body and flush cells.
- ➤ To recirculate health-promoting and immune-enhancing lymph fluid.
- ➤ To synchronize the sympathetic and parasympathetic nervous system.
- ➤ To align and balance the body. As the old saying goes, "You're only as old as your spine is." Yoga helps support posture, bringing the spine into alignment and creating more space and movement.
- ➤ To make you more conscious about yourself and your habits, including those that govern how you choose to eat. Studies have shown that yoga can help people automatically make better dietary decisions.

Sometimes, people avoid trying yoga because they think it's all about breathing or that it comes with many risks for injury. And some still hold on to false beliefs that yoga won't burn calories or stimulate weight loss. Much to the contrary, yoga confers multiple health benefits, ranging from stimulating the body's metabolic pathways to encouraging fat loss and muscle gain, to detoxifying tissues, lifting moods, increasing flexibility, improving cardiovascular health markers, inspiring creativity, and even tapping our most latent mental capabilities. According to William J. Broad, author of the illuminating, well-researched book *The Science of Yoga:* "There's been study after study after study that says you do not get your heart pumping in the way you do in aerobic sports like running, swimming and spinning. . . . On the other hand . . . yoga has this remarkable quality to relax you, to de-stress you. That means your heart rate goes down. That means if you're prone to hypertension, that lowers. There are all these wonderful cardio effects that come from the other end of the spectrum: the relaxation of the heart, rather than the pumping-up phenomena that you get from aerobic sports."

> *Additional idea: Pilates. If you've got a yoga practice in place or just want an alternative, try a Pilates class. This related exercise will afford you many of the same benefits of yoga, but uses a slightly different approach and setting. Group classes, mat Pilates, and one-on-one instruction using the Pilates Reformer machine are widely available today.*

I should also point out the sexual benefits that yoga can provide. Multiple studies have shown that yoga can prompt an increase in sex hormones. Which probably explains why recent studies in India looking at married couples who took up yoga revealed that, across the board, they experienced an improvement in desire, arousal, orgasm, and overall satisfaction. But, as Broad notes in his book, there is much about life that science cannot address, much less answer. He writes that many of yoga's truths surely go beyond the truths of science. And I have to agree.

Who benefits the most from yoga? Although all body types do, pitta types tend to more easily gravitate toward the practice since they are drawn to physically demanding activities. But pitta types need to be careful not to overdo it, just as kapha types should opt for more challenging forms of yoga than they may otherwise choose. And vata types should go for gentle yoga postures, especially sitting postures that can help them to ground their bodies and calm their minds.

Deep Breathing: Breathing exercises are par for the course in Ayurveda. According to ancient texts, breath is the single most important food. Indeed, it's a nutrient that we require to feed every cell with prana—life. According to Ayurveda, breath creates the fundamental connection between life, concrete matter, and intangible consciousness. It provides the network among body, mind, senses, and spirit.

We know that breathing is essential to life, but its benefits go far beyond just exchanging carbon dioxide waste for life-sustaining oxygen to the body. Slow, controlled breathing in particular is the foundation for an Ayurvedic way of life that aims to return the body to a more balanced state, and one that has removed signs of stress. When you're concentrating on your breathing, you create a shift in your mind that helps tame stressors, delivering you to a deeper level of awareness and consciousness. And let's not forget that deep breathing supports many healthful activities in the body. In addition to boosting the flow of oxygen throughout the body and brain (oxygen is probably the most critical ingredient for life; we would die within minutes without it), it benefits the immune system as well. Here's how: Lymph is a clear fluid filled with immune cells that moves around the body in a series of vessels that comprise the lymphatic system. Lymph is a linchpin of sorts to your immune system because it carries nutrients and collects cellular waste while helping to eradicate pathogens—including those that can antagonize a healthy metabolism and weight. The deeper you breathe, the more you can achieve this effect. It helps to think of the heart as the pump for the vascular system while your breaths and physical movement power up the lymphatic system, which has no built-in pump. Although we've long known that exercise stimulates the movement of lymphatic fluid, breathing's role wasn't identified until scientists could see lymph flow in lab studies. This is how we found out that deep breathing prompts the lymph to move through the lymphatic vessels.

> *Breathing is one of the most detoxifying actions of the body. Your body is designed to release a great majority of its toxins through breathing. The mere act of exhaling releases carbon dioxide—a natural waste of your body's metabolism—which has been passed from your bloodstream into your lungs.*

The nervous system, and, in particular, the sympathetic nervous system also benefit from deep breathing. If you live in today's hyperkinetic world, your sympathetic nervous system is probably overworked. This is the part of you that is sensitive to stress and anxiety, for it controls your fight-or-flight response and will trigger those surges in adrenaline and the stress hormone cortisol. We know that chronic stress depletes your body's nutrients and destabilizes your hormonal chemistry, which is partly why depression, muscle tension and pain, blood sugar imbalances, and GI issues are among the many conditions related to a sympathetic nervous system in overdrive. The good news? You can counteract this mechanism by triggering a relaxation response through the *parasympathetic* nervous system via deep breathing. It's the quickest means of getting these two systems to communicate. What you're essentially doing is flipping the switch from high alert to low as your heart rate slows, your muscles relax, and your blood pressure lowers. And all of this can happen in a matter of seconds.

Mastering the art of deep breathing is easy. Although there are various forms of deep breathing, some of which can plunge you into a meditative state, I won't get too complicated or fancy here (for additional ideas on breathing techniques and instructive videos, go to www.hotbellydiet.com). I merely want you to take two to three minutes twice daily during which you disengage from your work, close your eyes, and focus on taking a series of deep breaths. Inhale through your nose and fill your chest as you count to five. Once your lungs are filled, count to three and then exhale fully but slowly. Then repeat. As you do this exercise, you should feel your diaphragm move methodically up and down while you breathe in and out as your belly expands and contracts naturally. Schedule your twice-daily deep-breathing exercise just as you would schedule important appointments. Perhaps you can do one session upon waking as a way to start your day and do another session before heading home from work. It doesn't really matter when you do your deep breathing. Just aim to engage in two sessions a day; it'll take fewer than ten minutes total, but the payoffs are incalculable.

Bonus Work: Sweat It Out in Stationary Sweat Sessions

Sweating has an ancient history. The skin is the largest organ of your body, and a key participant in eliminating waste products just like the lungs. Because of its size and area, your skin actually removes more cellular waste than the colon and kidneys combined. Clearly, sweating occurs naturally during physical activity, which is why exercise has so many benefits from a detox perspective. But sweating can be induced through a sauna or steam bath, and although this type of sweating doesn't confer the exact same health rewards as the kind that accompanies physical exercise, it nevertheless offers many benefits that support vibrant health and weight maintenance.

First, sweat therapy releases toxins from the skin and at the same time relaxes muscles, easing aches and pains. Because so many toxins get expelled through perspiration, this essentially lessens the load on the kidneys and liver. Second, the use of a sauna or steam room raises your body's core temperature, which alone will aid the detox process. What's more, sweat therapy has also been shown to have a favorable impact upon the immune system, for it's one of the few known ways—in addition to sleep—to safely stimulate an increased production of growth hormone, which helps the body shed fat, revitalize cells, and support lean muscle mass. Sweat therapy also aids the autonomic nervous system, which governs muscle tension, heart rate and blood pressure, breathing and digestion, among other involuntary functions. I should also note that sweating often has the added effect of helping to control cravings and overeating. In Ayurveda, we say that when your body is overloaded with fat swirling around, it cannot breathe properly through your skin, as the pores become clogged. The result is feeling overheated, prompting you to seek food in an attempt to reduce the uncomfortable sensation. And one of the classical ways to open up those windows on the skin is through sweating; it will cool you down and regulate your metabolic function.

If you don't have access to a sauna or steam room, you can create a similar environment in your own bathroom with hot water from the shower or just by soaking in a hot bath until you sweat profusely. Or you can dress yourself in a sweat suit and go for a brisk walk (which clearly offers a combination of mild exercise and forced sweating). Try to schedule at least one sweat session a week. You may find it helpful to end your Sunday evening with a sweat therapy session in preparation for the new week ahead, as you purge out the old and welcome the new. One rule: Do any traditional workout routine before a stationary sweat session. In other words, get your exercise over and done with before entering a sauna or soaking in a hot tub.

Putting It All Together

I've given you a lot of information and ideas in this chapter. Please don't let it overwhelm you, much less inhibit you from getting out there and moving! Remember, my most basic wish for you is to add a walking routine to your day. You can start simply and build upon the foundation you create as you course through the Hot Belly Diet. By the time you reach Phase 3, my hope is that you've established a cardio base from which you can challenge yourself further. Try a new sport or a more advanced yoga class, or commit to a thirty- to sixty-minute daily exercise routine. Just be mindful of your limitations, and try not to overdo your workouts to the point you feel burned out and uninspired to keep going. Remember, the chief goals here are to increase circulation, improve blood flow, strengthen muscles, and create stability, flexibility, balance, and—perhaps most important—a higher sense of self-awareness. All of these can be achieved without feeling like you have to train for an Olympic event. You just need to move your body as frequently as possible throughout the day. Never strain or push the body to extremes. Adapt to the exercise of your choice as your body sees fit.

Below is a sample of how a typical week might look if you follow my guidelines. You'll see that I've called the weekend days "nature days." I encourage you to use the weekend to bring your workouts outdoors so you can commune with nature. Feel free to take one day off a week during which you don't engage in any exercise other than walking. This will give you the respite you need to start anew.

MONDAY	TUESDAY	WEDNESDAY	THURSDAY	FRIDAY	SATURDAY, SUNDAY
Thirty minutes formal cardio work	Yoga class	Thirty minutes formal cardio work	Yoga class	Thirty minutes formal cardio work	Nature days (e.g., a hike in the hills, a bicycle ride, a leisure walk)

For optimal results, log your exercise activities. It's long been proven that when we track our achievements, we're more likely to stick to our goals and be accountable for our intentions. You can track your progress the old-fashioned way using a pen and paper, or you can employ one of the many digital applications available today through the Internet or your smartphone. The mere act of logging your activities (and you can do this with your diet as well) will have an immediate effect on your level of consciousness—raising your awareness and attuning you to your world and environment in ways that can effortlessly support your weight-loss objectives and general health.

CHAPTER 8

The Hot Belly Diet and Disease Prevention

Let food be thy medicine, and medicine be thy food.

—HIPPOCRATES (460–377 BC)

I t's really true what they say about the relationship between health and lifestyle, which, of course, includes diet. As the old proverb goes, "With proper diet and lifestyle, medicine is of no need. With improper diet and lifestyle, medicine is of no use." Health, not illness, is our natural state. It's usually just a matter of finding it tucked beneath the layers of imbalance that have accumulated over time. In working toward a balanced body with a healthy metabolism, there's an important rule to remember: *Your body only wants to heal.* A human body is an individual organism that is self-manufactured, self-regenerating, and self-healing. When you cut your skin, your body immediately begins the mending process. When one of your body's organs or systems becomes aggravated or invaded by a germ, your body responds automatically with an elaborate series of brilliant, built-in mechanisms that know exactly what to do to restore health or, in some cases, kill the invader and then reestablish balance. But with repeated insults over time, this powerful balancing system can become overwhelmed and compromised. And what can result is disease, or "dis-ease," which literally means a lack of ease or balance. The good news is that even while enduring or fighting a major illness, the body still retains its natural inclination to heal. The key to activating and sustaining this healing potential rests in treating health with wholeness.

I'm a firm believer in the power of lifestyle, which commands whether or not you move closer to a revolving door of serial illness and physiological dysfunction or the achievement of a long, happy life free of serious ailments and ongoing conditions to manage. Unfortunately, many of us don't pay attention to imbalances until they reach the point of being painful or the symptoms can no longer be masked by medications. Take, for example, the mere experience of indigestion. You dismiss it initially and eventually reach for some antacids at meals because the burning sensation continues for several days or weeks. But then the pain starts to affect your sleep, and work becomes a challenge because of the exhaustion. So you go visit your doctor, who diagnoses a stomach ulcer that can luckily be treated.

The above scenario is one that millions go through. But those who are attuned to their dosha might be able to avert the doctor visit just by pausing to think about what's likely going on inside. The burning sensation in your stomach is a sign that pitta is out of balance. And if you're a pitta type by nature, you would know to make some shifts in your diet and eat more cooling, alkalizing foods to recover that balance again. You would also consider your overall mood and lifestyle. Are you stressed out? Overworked? If yes, then you would focus on engaging in more calming, stress-reducing activities. Those who are a vata or kapha type would also work on balancing pitta, but since these folks aren't naturally prone to overheating, they would do well to just soothe their stomachs after eating by choosing calming, cooling foods and liquids (e.g., coconut, cucumber, basmati rice, and herbal teas).

Today many of us suffer from chronic lifestyle diseases that are mostly attributed to how we choose to live. As I like to remind patients, you are not only *what* you eat, but also *when, why, how,* and *where*. And, as you've no doubt begun to understand since beginning this book, your eating habits are just a small piece of the equation, for you are also the outcome of your thoughts, emotions, and daily experiences.

This chapter offers you a respite from the instructive elements of the book's main program. Here is where I will immerse you in an absorbing lesson about the connection between diet/lifestyle and disease prevention, drawing from the latest in scientific research and describing how breakthroughs in physics and medicine are underscoring the validity of the five-thousand-year-old Ayurvedic medical system. The previous chapter already gave you a whirlwind tour of how we can marry Ayurvedic wisdom and modern medicine within the realm of exercise. Now, let's repeat the lesson on the parallels between ancient Indian science and today's Western perspective on disease.

Although we view our body as a physical mass or solid, it is in fact more like a fire that is constantly being renewed. Our cells turn over continually. This time next year, most of the total number of atoms in your body will have been replaced. Ayurveda essentially provides the tools to intervene at this quantum level. As I mentioned in the beginning of the book, Ayurveda tells us that freedom from illness and disease depends on bringing our own awareness into balance and then applying that balance to the body.

Building a Balanced Body in 21 Days

It's a question you might have been asking: Why did I design a 21-day Accelerate Phase for the core part of the Hot Belly Diet? After all, I could have just as easily formulated a ten-day or forty-day protocol. But that wouldn't have jibed well with either the science of

Ayurveda or the science of making a monumental change in your physiology. Not only do 21 days allow the body to create what's called a "cellular memory" so you can effortlessly maintain the weight loss, but we also derive 21 days from Ayurvedic math. We all know that nourishment from food is necessary for life. But how food actually fuels the body is often misunderstood. Ayurveda identifies seven vital tissues that provide the tools for the body's growth and structure. These tissues, called *dhatus,* are strikingly similar to the major tissues that modern science identifies, such as blood, muscle, fat, bone, and so on.

The building of tissues begins when food is digested. Starting with plasma, the tissues form layer by layer in a sequence. Muscle, for example, originates from both plasma and blood. The complexity of tissues increases with each new layer, culminating with the reproductive fluids. A problem or imbalance within any tissue will impact all subsequent tissues. Unhealthy plasma, for example, will affect all layers. Agni is at the heart of our body's tissue-building process through its role in helping sustain these vital tissues. A weak agni condition will result in the improper formation and maintenance of tissues. And the dhatus are integrally linked to an individual's

The Seven Dhatus

1. Plasma (*rasa*)
2. Blood (*rakta*)
3. Muscle (*mamsa*)
4. Fat (*meda*)
5. Bone (*asthi*)
6. Bone marrow and nerve (*majja*)
7. Reproductive fluid (*shukra/artava*)

dosha—one of three metabolic principles connecting the mind and body. Given the seven tissues and three doshas, we arrive at 21 days (seven times three); during this period, we are stimulating the proper metabolic flow within the body to burn energy and build healthy tissues. Hence, flow, burn, and build, or, as we say in Ayurvedic circles, prana, tejas, and ojas.

We all know that each of us is designed differently. We all may have very similar body parts and needs, but our individual features are strikingly unique, from our outward appearances to our inner workings, metabolisms, ways of thinking, personality, psyche . . . all the way down to our DNA. Ayurveda teaches that every health-related behavior, whether it's what we eat or how we exercise, must be evaluated in terms of each person's constitution. This contrasts with the Western approach, which focuses more on the properties of a medicine or the steps of a protocol rather than on the characteristics of the individuals for whom those treatments are prescribed.

Although it's a mental habit to separate our digestive system from all the others, it's uniquely tied to virtually every single cell, organ, and tissue in the body. Nutrients from foods we eat reach the deepest and most complex tissues. An ideal diet and perfectly functioning digestion ensure proper tissue renewal. But if the diet and digestion are less than perfect, then ama begins to build in each layer of tissue. The dhatus are connected to your individual doshic state. Just as balance within the doshas creates harmony in the tissues, imbalance foments disarray. If you have a dosha in excess, it will travel throughout the body and lodge itself in weak tissues and organs, where it can wreak havoc until balance is restored. We'll be exploring this concept shortly. First, let's gain a more modern understanding of why our power to heal rests largely with digestion.

The Power of Digestion: The Honest-to-Gut Truth

Hippocrates, who is often thought of as the father of modern Western medicine, could not have been more right when he sagely said that food and medicine go hand in hand. But it's quite amazing to think that only in the last decade have scientists revealed just how critical our digestion is to our overall health and well-being. It's our "second brain," in fact. And it's much bigger than the bundle of neurons inside your skull.

The role of digestion on health levels is sorely overlooked. Most people underestimate the importance of intestinal health. It's often easy to tolerate and disregard an occasional episode of heartburn or

Digesting Digestive Disorders

About ninety million people in the United States suffer from digestive disorders, from the occasional upset stomach, heartburn, or constipation to the more life-threatening diseases such as colorectal cancer. These conditions account for more than 104 million doctor visits per year and encompass disorders of the entire gastrointestinal tract, as well as the liver, gallbladder, and pancreas. Irritable bowel syndrome is thought to be the second leading cause of missed work, behind the common cold. Most digestive disorders are very complex, with subtle symptoms and unknown or vague causes. Although some have genetic roots, many develop from environmental and lifestyle factors such as chronic stress, fatigue, poor diet, sedentariness, and smoking. Alcohol abuse causes the greatest risk for digestive diseases.

diarrhea, but these ailments are far too common these days and are doing more health-depleting damage than we think. Put simply, a healthy digestion, or gut, acts as a center of gravity for all things health related. In fact, your digestive system is not just a processing plant for food; it's really the heart and soul of your entire immune system, as well as the defender of your overall well-being. Although we have many barometers today that we can use to tell us when something is wrong, such as blood pressure and heart rate, trouble with weight and any existing digestive disorders are a quick and easy telltale sign of the body experiencing an imbalance.

We have a tendency to link illness and disease to certain germs or specific organs of the body without even thinking about how our guts may have played a role in that illness. Or we focus on the organs that seem to have more of an immediate impact on whether or not we survive for another minute, such as our hearts that have to continue beating, or our brains that must keep firing neurons. We can't go more than a few minutes or even seconds without a heartbeat or active brain waves, yet we can last for several days without food or water.

More than anything, it helps to think of digestion as your body's primary energy assembly line, organizer, and orchestrator. It's the front lines of our survival. And it must be working properly for everything else in the body to be on cue. Not only is your digestive system arguably the most important ingredient in your overall health and weight equation, but it's also intimately involved in your emotional, intuitive side. Think about it: We rely upon our "gut instinct" or "gut feeling" to tell us the right thing to do. We talk about our "gut reactions," and fall prey to nausea and butterflies in our stomach when we're nervous, excited, or scared. We "follow our guts" or do a "gut check" when encountering a big decision. And we refer to our guts within the context of courage and fortitude (i.e., "has guts").

This is not an arbitrary connection we like to make between our guts and our real brain. Thanks to some remarkable research performed in the past decade, we know that the digestive system—the gut—is synced up with the brain in seemingly unimaginable ways. Indeed, your gut and your "first brain" housed in your head communicate seamlessly through an intimate, two-way connection. Every class of neurochemical produced in the first brain is also manufactured in the gut, including those that relate directly with mood and well-being. In fact, your gut's brain makes more serotonin, which is the master happiness molecule, than the brain that rests in your head. An estimated 80 to 90 percent of the total amount of serotonin in your body is manufactured by the nerve cells in your gut!

We tend to put much more importance on the brain in our head than the complex network of nerve cells and neurotransmitters that operate in our intestines. But it's true: This beautiful orchestra of nerves in our gut can process information and generate responses just like our head's brain. So stunningly complex is this relationship that the digestive tract can be considered the largest sensory organ in the body. Recent research is revealing that perhaps our second brain may not be "second" at all. It can act separate from the main brain and independently control many functions without the main brain's input or help. The gut actually directs its own little network that allows it to respond to the brain and initiate signals when something isn't right. This process ensures that the digestive system is continually harmonizing with your overall state. In addition to nerve signals, the gut also sends out hormonal signals that reach the brain directly or through stimulation of the sensory nerves. Certain intestinal hormones, for instance, can transmit sensations of fullness and hunger. Similarly, when inflammation is underway somewhere in the digestive tract, the intestines can also send a message to the brain that conveys sensations such as pain, fatigue, the need for more sleep, and a feeling of illness. Put another way, if you suffer from an illness or infection that impacts your digestion, how you feel will be a factor of your gut's influences on your brain and can even have an impact on your thoughts, level of pain, sleep, and level of energy.

It is because the digestive system sends an enormous amount of information to an area of the brain responsible for our self-awareness and sense of well-being that it's such a prominent player in our perception of health and wellness. In fact, improving the relationship between our brain and our digestion can improve everything about us—mentally, physically, and emotionally. The scientists who study this amazing brain-gut link stress the importance of eating a healthy diet and avoiding oversized, high-calorie, difficult-to-digest, heavy meals, particularly when eaten late at night as our digestion enters its fasting mode. Otherwise, one can experience intestinal disturbances that further lead to feelings of distress.

No Bugging Around

We can't talk about a healthy gut without considering our friends that help the process. I'm referring to the bacteria that fill your intestinal tract and that participate in your digestion, metabolism, and overall health. Within the body of a healthy adult, microbial cells are estimated to outnumber human cells by a factor of ten to one. Each person shelters about ten times the number of microbes than cells. They assist in the digestion of some vitamins and they play a significant role in our immune system. For the most part, though, these microbial cells (bacteria, fungi such as yeast, and viruses) remain largely unstudied. Recently, the NIH launched the Human Microbiome Project (HMP; you can learn more at www.hmpdacc .org) with the mission of understanding the influence of microbes upon human development, physiology, immunity, and nutrition so we can characterize the human microbiota (the microbe population in our guts, often referred to as the microbiome or intestinal flora) within the realm of human health and disease. In 2013, for instance, studies began to emerge showing a stunning connection between the state of our guts' ecosystem and the risk for one of the most dreaded diseases of all: cancer. The headline said it all: "What if a key factor ultimately behind a cancer was not a genetic defect but ecological?" No joke: The gut is like a rain forest—an intricate ecosystem constantly at the mercy of changes in its environment.

From a very broad standpoint, our bodies perform two fundamental physiological jobs. First, we assimilate nutrients, and, second, we expel waste products of that energy metabolism through several channels such as the colon, lungs, and sweat glands. Everyday physiological processes like energy production, digestion, and hormone synthesis generate waste products that can interfere with the body's functionality if they aren't neutralized or disposed of. But our intestinal microbiota also produce waste, and we can harbor good, bad, and neutral colonies. (There are microbes in other areas of our body as well, such as the skin microbiota that could play into psoriasis, and the urogenital microbiota that can factor into reproductive and sexual diseases.)

The good bacteria are often called "probiotics" (a term that means "for life") because of the role they play in keeping us healthy. These gut-friendly cohabitants make substances that help to destroy harmful bacteria. *Lactobacillus acidophilus* and *Bifidobacteria bifidum* are just two prominent examples of these beneficial bacteria that are often found in fortified yogurt. Examples of bad flora include salmonella and *Candida albicans,* a yeast that can cause an infection when it grows out of control. Bad flora are constantly taking in nutrients and creating wastes that often result in gas and bloating. If internal toxins are not brought under control, over the long term they can contribute to a weakened immune system, inflammation, and a slower metabolic rate. Obviously, we want the good bacteria to be more prevalent than the bad bacteria. We can't ever eradicate all the bad bacteria, for they are a part of life. But if the balance is upset, we see an increased risk for myriad health issues.

Your gut is your body's first line of defense. You know this because when a nasty microbe is mistakenly consumed, the gut quickly recognizes the intruder and leaps into action. But to identify the culprit, it must call upon millions of immune system cells residing in its walls that are at the ready for war. For this reason, as I mentioned, the gut is a major player in immunity, helping to differentiate between what is harmless and what is harmful. Every day, your gut encounters pounds of foreign material in the form of sustenance. The immune system is like a gatekeeper; it has to decide what is okay to let through and what is not. And it doesn't like to be fooled.

This extraordinary system gets going the day you enter the world. At birth, your gastrointestinal tract was entirely free of bacteria, but moments thereafter it began to be colonized. And during the first few years of life, your gut developed a unique tribe of bacterial species whose characteristics were determined by a variety of factors, including genetics, diet, hygiene, geography, medication use, and even the tribes of bacteria colonizing people around you. And because these microbes take up residence on the delicate folds of your intestinal walls, they help create a physical barrier against potential invaders such as bad bacteria (pathogenic flora), viruses, and parasites. The intestinal flora also have a role in preventing infections and combating many toxins that make it down into your intestines. The good bacteria also digest part of your food. Just as microorganisms in the soils of a forest help break down fallen fruit to return nutrients to the plants and trees, your gut's microorganisms are charged with aiding in the extraction of essential nutrients from foods so that they can be absorbed across the intestinal wall and into the bloodstream for delivery to cells and tissues. Without these bacteria, you'd be at a loss for transporting many nutrients, which explains why a depletion of healthy gut flora pretty much guarantees nutrient depletion and its consequences, system malfunction. Anyone who has taken antibiotics and experienced gastrointestinal issues as a result knows what happens when you wipe out your gut's friendly bacteria.

Suddenly, you're missing an important part to your body's healthy functionality.

We in fact rely on our gut's flora to absorb certain nutrients, some as important as the B vitamins. Without these nutrients being predigested by bacteria, we simply cannot absorb them. It is becoming known that fermented foods are beneficial to our health. Fermentation is another way of saying "predigested by bacteria." The intestinal flora acts as a fermentation tank inside our gut. Functionally, it becomes an auxiliary organ of digestion, detoxifying up to

Your Inner Ecology

As reported in *ScienceDaily*, a key factor behind cancerous growth could very well be the ecological damage found in our gut:

> Ecologists have long known that when some major change disturbs an environment in some way, ecosystem structure is likely to change dramatically. Further, this shift in interconnected species' diversity, abundances, and relationships can in turn have a transforming effect on the health of the whole landscape—causing a rich woodland or grassland to become permanently degraded, for example—as the ecosystem becomes unstable and then breaks down the environment. . . .

And, indeed, it is for this reason that any disturbance in the body can dramatically change its community of collaborators in health, including those colonies of bacteria that have a huge say in whether we are healthy or not (and can lose or gain weight). And such changes can lead to unexpected and significant adverse effects.

40 percent of the toxins it comes in contact with in your food. In other words, when you kill the good bacteria in your gut, which can be done through an imbalanced diet, you are almost doubling the workload of your digestive tract and related organs like the liver. Perhaps your microbiome's most important job, however, is to stimulate and maintain the body's immune system. Through its multiple functions in the digestive tract, your microbiome dictates a lot about your health and ability to prevent, manage, and cure disease.

New research shows that the microbes in healthy people are much more diverse from site to site than previously thought, and also from person to person. Scientists have learned that the specific bacteria at a site are less important than the functions they perform. Nobody really knows what right combination of species is the ideal one for an individual. We are just beginning to tap into the understanding of what goes on in healthy guts, and even more recently into how micro-organisms in our gut are associated with many more problems than we ever thought. But one thing is certain: The specific microbial tribe you develop and harbor has a big say in your health. In addition to fortifying your resistance to disease, the population of microbes in your gut may lower your risk of a medley of disorders and diseases. Researchers are currently looking at the possible role that some strains of intestinal bacteria have in obesity, inflammatory and functional GI disorders, chronic pain, autism, depression, and autoimmune disorders such as rheumatoid arthritis, multiple sclerosis, and psoriasis. Scientists are also examining the role that these bacteria play in our emotions. Maybe we'll discover one day that a certain strain of bacteria or community of microbes in the digestive system can foretell whether someone is generally happy and optimistic, or depressive and pessimistic.

One overarching feature that studies on the microbiome are revealing is the diversity of bacteria in the human body, akin to a rain forest. Different regions of the body are home to different combinations of species. No two people are "growing" alike. I could have an

The Health in Hormones

Since the beginning of this book, I've been referring to hormones in passing and suggesting that their balanced flow through the body plays into our health and wellness. I cannot overstate this enough: Our collective basket of hormones, the endocrine system, holds the remote control to much of what we feel—moody, tired, hungry, sexual, sick, healthy, hot, or cold. Our endocrine system lords over development, growth, reproduction, and behavior through an intricate system of hormones, which are the body's chemical messengers. Most of these messengers are manufactured in one part of the body (e.g., the thyroid, adrenal, or pituitary gland or gonads) and pass into the bloodstream to reach target organs and tissues. It helps to think of hormones as traffic signs and signals; they tell your body what to do so it can run smoothly. Besides managing your reproductive system, they serve a vital role in every bodily system, including your urinary, respiratory, cardiovascular, nervous, muscular, skeletal, immune, and digestive systems.

And when hormones become imbalanced, you will notice it either by a subtle sense that something isn't right or through a bona fide diagnosis (and the potential diagnoses affiliated with hormones are many: metabolic and thyroid disorders, infertility, cancer, chronic pain, hair loss, fatigue, a loss of libido, and depression). Hormonal chaos can happen quite naturally during stressful periods or as a result of your age and various health conditions that disrupt the harmony. Or they can become imbalanced under the influence of toxins that interfere with the body's innate hormonal machinery. The good news is that hormonal dysfunction can often be addressed *through the diet* . . . and through a plan of action outlined by the Hot Belly Diet. As you gain control of your digestive powers, you will notice that the emanating wellness in your belly will have profound, positive effects on your entire endocrine system.

entirely different colony of bacteria thriving in my body than you, which affects whether or not my diet helps me to maintain a healthy digestive system. In the future, perhaps I'll know enough about my unique type of microbiome to keep my digestive system running as smoothly as possible. Within the next ten years, researchers will uncover mysteries of the microbiome and begin to find ways in which we can manipulate it to support health. And I have no doubt that these findings will dovetail what Ayurveda has been teaching for centuries about the relationship between one's personal constitution and one's capacity to achieve optimal health.

The Six Stages of Disease

Very few of us wake up with a sudden, serious illness. We're more likely to endure repeated blows that trigger a massive biological imbalance over time. It is the continual excess of certain foods, activities, emotions, or ways of thinking that triggers the disease process. Ayurveda sees health as a dynamic process, not a static state. Likewise, disease is an equally dynamic process with many factors leading up to the ultimate insult of a bona fide diagnosis that Western medicine will then try to treat.

One of the main goals of medicine that is not unique to Ayurveda is putting people back in touch with their own nature. This is also true for practitioners of Western medicine, even though it prefers physical explanations for disease that can be proven through the rigors of the scientific method. But Western medicine has made some concessions in recent times, finally agreeing that disease can just as easily originate in the mind as in the body (hence the newly sprung term "mind-body medicine"). It's well documented, for instance, that people who suffer a traumatic loss, such as the death of a spouse, are highly vulnerable to sudden death from a heart attack. But when pressed to explain the connection, doctors are forced to rely more on vague notions about the power of emotions in controlling master switches in the body's physiology than on any particular biochemical or physical defect. In fact, the interaction between the mind and the body (and its immune system) is so fluid, intangible, and complex that modern medicine still cannot explain exactly when certain triggers, such as poor diet or negative thoughts, compromise the body's health and normal operating system. Ayurveda, on the other hand, can be a little more precise.

According to ancient texts, the disease process can be broken down into six distinct stages—accumulation, aggravation, spreading or dissemination, localization, manifestation, and differentiation. The first three are usually invisible and can be linked to either the body or the mind. The last three typically entail overt symptoms that you and your doctor can identify or that can be detected with technology. Each stage reflects a loss of balance, a departure from the body's natural workings. Let me describe these stages in detail, giving you a different, but compelling new way to understand, appreciate, and ultimately prevent illness. This will in turn reinforce not just the power of digestion, but the role that nourishment (i.e., food choices) plays in health and wellness. In my world, I try to treat imbalances at their earliest stage, and it goes without saying that the foods we eat are integral components in all six stages.

Stage 1: Accumulation

In this first stage of disease, minor symptoms begin to emerge that you may not even notice initially or you ignore the slight discomfort. This is when one or more doshas (pitta, kapha, or vata) becomes aggravated and then begins to build up. Ideally, you notice the imbalance in an innate urge to correct it somehow. So, to offer a very primitive but illustrative example, let's say you've been eating cold ice cream daily after dinner. After a week, you feel sluggish and another bowl of ice cream doesn't feel appetizing anymore. Instead, you crave

Your Dosha Dictionary

Each dosha has a principle location or "seat." Kapha's seat is in the chest. Pitta's seat is in the small intestine. Vata's seat is in the colon. When a dosha starts to go out of balance, the first signs will often occur at its seat. For example, intestinal problems such as bloating, gas, and constipation are signs of an aggravated vata; a mad pitta can manifest in a hot or painful sensation in the upper abdomen; and a head cold, cough, or chest congestion signals an aggravated kapha. This doesn't go to say that the first symptoms of imbalance always show up in these sites. A vata imbalance can hide in other parts of the lower abdomen, disclosing itself as menstrual cramps or lower back pain. Remember: Every dosha is present in all parts of the body, and dosha imbalances can migrate or show up as mysterious conditions in areas of the body far from their original seat. That said, viewing illness within the context of dosha imbalances allows for more precise preventive tactics, especially when you know your body type's particular strengths and weaknesses based on its dominant dosha or essential nature.

Below is a cheat sheet you can use to understand dosha imbalances and innate tendencies based on particular doshas.

- *Vata* is unbalanced when there is pain, cramps, chills, spasms, or shakiness. Vata types are susceptible to insomnia, anxiety disorders, depression, chronic constipation, nervous stomach, cramps, irritable bowel, chronic pain, high blood pressure, and arthritis.

- *Pitta* is unbalanced when there is inflammation, fever, heartburn, hot flashes, or excessive hunger and thirst. Pitta types are vulnerable to heart disease, acne, heartburn, peptic ulcers, rashes, premature balding and gray hair, poor eyesight, hostility, and self-criticism.

- *Kapha* is unbalanced when there is congestion, mucus, discharge, fluid retention, lethargy, heaviness, or over-sleeping. Kapha types are prone to obesity, diabetes, high cholesterol, congested sinuses, chest colds, painful joints, asthma and/or allergies, depression, and feelings of slug-gishness in the morning.

Bear in mind that these relationships are not finite, deterministic, or prophetic. Just because you're a kapha type doesn't mean you'll die of diabetes. Likewise, a pitta type isn't doomed to have a heart attack. Nor does being one type protect you from the common ills of another type. Illness depends on a lot of factors, including your overall lifestyle patterns, and is highly individual. Although a body type can clue us in to important influences, it's not a causal element. Keep in mind, too, that most major disorders and diseases (e.g., heart disease, cancer) are the result or more than one dosha becoming imbalanced. When one is aggravated, the others follow suit if the imbalance persists. But knowing which dosha triggers the entire cascade of events can help you to nip the imbalance in the bud, so to speak.

just a fresh peach or other light fruit. This is your body telling you to seek balance. And by listening to this "inner intelligence," you can halt a disease process at the source. This is another reason why incorporating all six tastes into your diet as much as possible is important.

Stage 2: Aggravation

Once a disease process commences, the imbalanced dosha remains, continues to accumulate, and symptoms get worse. A pitta imbalance with an upset stomach, for example, can lead to acid indigestion during Stage 2, especially if pitta-provoking foods are consumed to further fan the flames. This is when the imbalanced dosha can begin to move elsewhere in the body and find a place where ama is present, to which it becomes stuck. The key to stopping Stage 2 from progressing to Stage 3 is to pay attention to dietary and lifestyle factors and make the appropriate adjustments to return to a state of balance (what traditional science would call "homeostasis"). For most people, this means shifting to a lighter diet that's easy on digestion, drinking dosha-balancing herbal teas, and easing up on dinners (or skipping them entirely). The most common ways that doshas become provoked during this stage are when vata types don't get enough rest, pitta types drink too much alcohol or eat too many spicy foods, and kapha types fail to get enough exercise.

Stage 3: Spreading or Dissemination

At this point, a disease has progressed and spilled into general circulation, reaching other areas of the body. As a result, symptoms slowly and subtly emerge in other parts of the body unrelated to the original source of the problem. But as with the first two stages, this one can be largely invisible to someone who is not paying attention. A classic example: Let's say you are on the verge of insulin resistance due to chronic blood-sugar imbalances. You have no idea what's going on at a cellular, hormonal level, but you notice that your cravings become insatiable, weight control becomes challenging, and you have a general lack of energy. Because these secondary symptoms are relatively minor and inconsistent, it's easy to disregard them or discredit them as serious. You go about your life and avoid thinking about the growing problem, although somewhere in the back of your mind you worry about what's going on, and you may even make futile attempts to watch what you eat. But this is when it's critical to intervene before disease continues to progress. In Ayurveda, methods of detoxification such as fasting and cleansing are highly recommended in addition to correcting dietary misdeeds fueling the imbalance. It's also important to identify lifestyle patterns that could have triggered and sustained the imbalance.

Stage 4: Localization

A disease in the localization stage is one in which the imbalanced dosha is permitted to camp out or "localize" in areas of the body where it doesn't belong, typically lodging itself in weak organs and systems throughout the body. What constitutes a weakness? Any number of things, ranging from a genetic predisposition to an infection or illness, to addiction, unresolved emotions, and external germs or pathogens that enter the body. Once the overpowering dosha combines with the tissues, a functional imbalance at a cellular level sets in. Most of us in this stage are aware of a problem now, no matter how much we tried to turn a blind eye or treat it on the surface with over-the-counter meds. If the condition is not dealt with here, a firm diagnosis is inevitable, and the disease becomes all the more difficult to manage or cure. Clearly, Stage 4 often entails the input of a medical professional who can help identify (diagnose) and treat the condition in pursuit of returning the body to a balanced, healthy state. Although traditional drugs could be part of the protocol at this juncture, dietary and lifestyle guidance is also recommended. The goal is to pacify the imbalanced dosha, cleanse the tissues of impurities, eliminate ama, and stimulate agni.

Stage 5: Manifestation

People in waiting rooms at doctor's offices (or in the emergency room) are likely in this stage, in which the symptoms are serious and undeniable. In the manifestation stage, the overwhelming dosha is prominent in the tissues and a combination of addressing the symptoms medically and restoring the health of the tissues through purification therapies is in order. This is when breaking poor dietary habits becomes absolutely essential, focusing on eating foods that will balance out the doshas and avoiding anything that will contribute to the accumulation of ama and more complications from the condition.

Stage 6: Differentiation

No one wants to get to this stage, which is also called "chronic" or "disruptive." In this final stage, the disease process is fully manifested, and specific symptoms have been labeled such that they point to a diagnosis that must be treated. Examples include type 2 diabetes, coronary artery disease, and rheumatoid arthritis. For some, the disease process can be reversed. But for many, it cannot and must now be carefully monitored and managed. In addition to using Western medicine, Ayurvedic principles will further help one get a handle on the disease process and limit its impact on the body and mind. These principles include detoxification measures and attention to dietary and lifestyle factors. Stage 6 often encompasses structural changes and negative impacts to other organs, so those must also be considered and addressed in the treatment plan. Once the disease process is under proper control, rejuvenating therapies through the diet can be used to rebuild and strengthen the tissues. This, in turn, can help assuage the condition's severity and overall effect on the body, including its longevity.

Even if you find yourself entering the latter stages of a disease's course, it doesn't mean that death looms large or that you're doomed to a lifetime of misery. Most everyone over the age of forty or forty-five experiences vague aches and pains that can cut into one's quality of life and spark tremendous, unnecessary worry. Our body is subjected to dietary, behavioral, and emotional imbalances through the years by virtue of life! So the more years you have behind you, the more likely you'll experience periodic imbalances. This is the reality of aging. What your body is telling you when you enter the latter stages is that you need to do two simple things: (1) pay attention, and (2) purify your tissues of excess doshas. Don't let negative thinking that you're in grave danger aggravate your imbalanced state further. You'd be amazed by how easily you can regain your natural balance—and put vata, pitta, and kapha back in their place—just by making a few fundamental shifts in diet and daily routine. And that's what the Hot Belly Diet is all about.

The Illness in Industrialized Foods

It's well understood now that we live in a world of processed and manufactured food. In my view, our modern eating habits have spurred many preventable health conditions as well as warped our sense of taste. I once consulted with Frito-Lay on creating a new flavor. My consulting ended when I learned that it wasn't enough to combine natural spices and ingredients, which could easily make for a delicious, mouthwatering seasoning on chips. The company needed to have a proprietary blend, one that contained a patented chemical. It's sad to think that from a young age today, our tongues are trained to eat chemicals that dupe our natural senses.

The body operates a vast network of not just sensory organs, but also transportation channels called "*srotas*." These consist of gross channels like the gastrointestinal tract, lymphatic system, urinary tract, and circulatory system, and the less tangible channels such as metabolic reactions and energetic pathways. The srotas are the avenues through which the doshas, dhatus, and so-called *malas* move throughout the body. Malas refer to waste products and include not just urine and feces, but sweat, mucus, tears, and ear wax and other oily secretions. All of these malas are related to some tissue. As I indicated in the last chapter, sweat is regarded as a waste product of fat. Mucus is similarly seen as a waste product of plasma. Although we may look upon these waste products in a negative manner, they are fundamental in the body's inherent cleansing, toning, and purifying functions. Without the efficient removal of malas, we'd be in all kinds of physiological trouble.

Since malas should find their exit, Ayurveda identifies thirteen natural urges that should not be resisted. They are: urination, defecation, hunger, thirst, a desire for sex, burping, vomiting, yawning, sneezing, passing gas, coughing, crying, and sleeping. Ayurveda also endorses the avoidance of three additional activities that we may find ourselves inclined to do, and they are: working beyond our capacity; unhealthy (negative) thinking, talking, and doing; and possessing negative emotions such as anger, greed, desire, addiction, fear, worry, and jealousy.

Imbalances with the doshas typically lead to the inability to effectively eliminate waste materials. And one of the most common ways imbalances occur is through diet alone. Initial symptoms can be as innocuous as a slight bloated feeling, but can develop into a serious, potentially life-threatening condition whereby impurities (substances toxic to the body) are reabsorbed and circulated throughout the body.

Without question, a healthy digestive system hinges on having clear, smoothly running channels that deliver nutrients while collecting and eliminating waste products. Any blockages in the srotas will inhibit these functions and render the body vulnerable to illness or injury. The srotas are the chief target areas for ama accumulation. And as ama builds in these channels, the body's transportation system is greatly compromised. Which is why maintaining good digestion is a crucial key to avoiding such obstructions. Taking one more step back, we can add that excellent digestion starts with good nutrition (*ahem:* as in less industrialized foods and more natural, vibrant, light, and *digestible* choices).

Honor Your Body's Intelligence

When I first saw Monica, she looked ten years older than her forty-something age. As a yoga instructor with her own studio, she taught four ninety-minute classes a day, which meant she had no time to eat properly. Monica may have had the super-skinny body of a model, but her face told another story—it was dry, heavily creased, and deeply wrinkled. She didn't sleep well at night, always woke up tired, and worried constantly about money and her business. She spent most of her day grumpy and irritated, despite the effects that yoga was supposed to be having on her! Her concerns over money prevented her from hiring more yoga instructors, so she could rest up.

I was blunt with my prescription for her: I told her that her studio was killing her and suggested that she close it for a month to focus on her health. Though she didn't shut down her studio (she gave the keys to someone who could take over), she did take the steps with me to change her life. We began by rekindling her fire, which had been left to smolder. Because she had shrunk her stomach down so much with her skimpy eating habits, her digestion had become grossly weak. Every time she ate, she experienced gas and bloating. But slowly over time, we got her system back up and running. For a month she avoided exercise and took to walking on the beach. By the second month, she looked totally different. Now she looked five years *younger* than her real age, and boasted a full, radiant face—not the shrunken prune of her previous life. Today she teaches one yoga class in the morning and one at night. And her business has taken off thanks to a new marketing strategy and a new sense of self.

Although Monica was seemingly doing "everything right" as a health-conscious yoga instructor, she was actually doing everything wrong for her body by not listening to it and responding to its needs. Today it's common for people to "forget" how to tune in to their bodies and practice what's called "self-referral"—referring to your ability to understand how you are feeling in every given situation and respond accordingly. After all, we now have gadgets and apps to help us determine how many calories we've burned and tell us what we should be eating. We tend to reach for food when we're really just thirsty. Most of us don't know when it's time to stop eating. To achieve a fit and healthy body, we must listen to what it's telling us. Ayurveda is a consciousness-based approach to health—it connects you to a higher awareness of yourself. We can't treat the body like a dumb machine and then expect it to take care of us. We need to take care of it and respect it. And tuning in to your inner intelligence is easier than you think!

If I were to ask you where the mind is located, what would you say? It's quite intuitive to think of the physical brain and its inner "intelligence," but the mind is found throughout the entire body. Our ability to think, reason, plan, calculate, perceive, and feel may be rooted in the consciousness of the mind, but we cannot say for certain that that "mind" is only found in the tangle of neurons that make up the physical brain. Indeed, the brain is the primary organ through which our mind functions, but it's not confined to the brain per se. A stream of consciousness and intelligence flows throughout the entire body—and through every cell. We call this the "nonlocalized mind," and the source of this stream is the same universal life force that I've been talking about. It's what creates the link between mind and body. It's also why we can be so affected by our thoughts and emotions. Feelings of joy, anger, fear, or anxiety can have physical manifestations. Physical disease almost always has a mental and emotional component; and untreated mental disease usually manifests in the physical body. This has been well documented by modern medicine, as clinical relationships have been confirmed between a variety of psychological issues and certain conditions. Just consider the basket of illnesses that chronic stress has been linked to: everything from panic anxiety disorder to heart disease and even cancer. And based on this indelible mind-body connection, we can further say that the entire body can be viewed as a dynamic, pulsating mind.

So, the question remains: How can you honor your body's intelligence to keep all of its cylinders firing? Let's turn to my twenty-one tips. These will help you to further live up to the Hot Belly Diet's lessons and the core principles of Ayurveda.

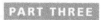

PART THREE

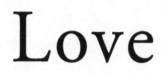

Love

CHAPTER 9

Twenty-One Tips to Maximizing and Maintaining Your Weight Loss

One whose doshas are balanced, whose tissues and wastes are functioning normally, whose appetite is good, and whose body, mind, and sense remain filled with bliss is called a healthy person.

—SUSHRUTA SAMHITA

The word "lifestyle" means something different to everyone. For some, lifestyle is about the way you live in terms of your geography, what you do for a living, and how you spend money and occupy leisure time. For others, lifestyle is more precisely about the choices you make daily in your routines, such as how you eat, when you sleep, and what you do for exercise and pure pleasure. Some may even include how they love, think, share with others, and search for purpose on this planet. However you describe "lifestyle," one thing is certain: It's not all about material goods or even outward, tangible signs of lifestyle; it's about our behavioral patterns that reflect our attitudes, beliefs, innermost thoughts, and general approach toward life. It's also about the relationships we keep *within ourselves* and about ourselves.

As you've learned by now, Ayurveda places prime importance on the connection between health and lifestyle, and the bond we continually have with nature. Health is not defined by numbers, measurements, and other metrics used by traditional Western medicine. Neither is the achievement of health relegated to counting calories, grams of fat, and time spent on a treadmill. Rather, health should be seen as a vastly more complex, intimate, and ever-changing experience that we enjoy when we're in balance with our inner constitution and the world at large. This is when our cells operate beautifully according to their inherent intelligence and we are able to tap that intrinsic wisdom to inform smart decisions about how to live.

Another key theme to Ayurveda that I've been instilling in you since the beginning of this book is that, despite some of the hype perpetuated by the modern media, the body doesn't naturally gravitate toward illness and disease even in advanced age. Health resides within all of us. Let me repeat that by stating this fact another way: The human body only wants to heal. I know that I mentioned this before, but it bears repeating. Health, not illness, is our natural state. So when we find ourselves sick or derailed somehow by a condition, it's not that health has totally escaped us. Illness doesn't take the place of health or expel it from our body. Much to the contrary, it helps to see health as always there—it's an omnipotent, ever-present part of us that can be eclipsed or masked by layers of imbalance that have accumulated over time. Which means it's often possible to find health again when we commit to supporting the body's natural healing potential and treating health with wholeness.

I've already given you ideas for improving your body's "health," especially with regard to boosting its weight-loss powers and rekindling its deep sources of physiological and metabolic renewal. Now, in this chapter, I'm going to highlight my twenty-one tips that further underscore my ideas and will help you to live up to the chief principles of an Ayurvedic lifestyle. Some of these may sound familiar to you because a few have been mentioned in passing. But here I will go into more details and hopefully cement these concepts into your brain so you don't forget them. My goal is not to reiterate typical weight-loss ideas that you've probably read about elsewhere, such as "preplan your meals," "create shopping lists," and "shop the perimeter of a grocery store," where most of the wholesome natural foods are found; instead, these ideas reflect more significant lifestyle habits that relate directly or indirectly to health and weight loss. Although you may wonder how, say, working on your relationships plays into your quest for a smaller waistline, you'd be surprised by how powerful these tips can be in helping you to achieve your goals—whatever they may be. Earlier, I talked about the importance of balancing what's called the shreyas and preyas. As a reminder, shreyas refers to what's eternally good for us, whereas preyas refers to that which is purely sensorial and mental and may not always be good for us. In Ayurveda, we say that shreyas are like good habits—they are hard to develop, but easy to live with; preyas, on the other hand, are like bad habits—they are easy to develop, but hard to live with. We also say that the habits you keep, and the habits you don't keep, will determine almost everything you achieve and fail to achieve in life.

I encourage you to incorporate as many of these tips into your life as possible. Make them habits you keep to the best of your ability. If you come across any that you just don't think are possible right now, that make you feel uncomfortable, or that won't work with your current chosen lifestyle, then skip them and move on to others. This isn't meant to be a laundry list of rigid to-dos. It's only meant to offer practical strategies for fulfilling that elusive goal of health that will work with every body type. You, however, are still in charge, and you inhabit a unique body. At the heart of my message is the importance of knowing yourself, as I am giving you the tools for raising your self-awareness so you can spot imbalances on the horizon before reaching and realizing them. Even if you just abide by some of these ideas, you will nonetheless reap enormous benefits and likely feel results sooner rather than later. It goes without saying that you don't need to do much to reinforce the body's instinctive proclivity toward health and optimal wellness. You are an incredibly self-regulating machine, even with regard to weight balance and the achievement of a perfect metabolism for you and your body. So take a moment to appreciate—and perhaps marvel at—that wondrous reality. And then open yourself to the possibilities that await you.

Tip #1: Schedule Your Sleep: Our bodies metabolize waste products mostly after 10:00 p.m.; this activity is reduced during wakeful, active hours. Moreover, the immune system needs to revitalize itself between 11:00 p.m. and 2:00 a.m., so it's critical to be asleep during these hours. It also helps to keep a rigid sleeping schedule 365 days a year.

Every day our bodies go through biological cycles tied to outward cues from nature. We all maintain a biological clock, or a circadian rhythm that entails patterns of repeated activity related to cycles of day and night—patterns that recur every twenty-four hours and are somehow synched with the solar day. This includes not only our sleep-wake cycle, but also the rise and fall of body temperature, and the ebb and flow of certain biochemicals and enzymes that dictate our physiology. Our body temperature rises during the day, peaks in the evening, then begins to go down again (it also takes a slight dip in the early afternoon, which brings on that late-day lull). A healthy day/night cycle makes for healthy hormonal release patterns, from those associated with our eating habits to those that relate to restful sleep, immunity, and cellular recovery. Our chief appetite hormones, ghrelin and leptin, for example, orchestrate the yin and yang of our eating patterns, essentially telling us when we're hungry and when we've had enough. The science that has made these digestive hormones so popular lately is breathtaking: We have proof now that inadequate sleep creates an imbalance of both hormones, which in turn affects hunger and appetite. In one well-cited study, when people slept just four hours a night for two consecutive nights, they experienced a 24 percent increase in the consumption of high-calorie treats, salty snacks, and starchy foods. The lesson: Sleep deprivation essentially disrupts the connection from our brain to our stomach; it fools our body into thinking it's hungry when it's not and coaxes us to gravitate toward foods that can spoil a healthy diet. Hence the term *mindless eating*.

Cortisol, a key hormone in the body that's involved with many important physiological processes, including metabolism, immune function, and blood pressure regulation, should be at its highest levels in the morning and progressively decrease throughout the day, dipping to its lowest levels after 11:00 p.m., at which point another hormone, melatonin, surges. Melatonin is our body's natural sleep

---

Sleep Is Vital

The quality and amount of sleep you get has an astonishing impact on virtually every system in your body. Just a generation ago, we didn't think much about the value of sleep other than to refresh our body to some degree. Today, however, the study of sleep constitutes an entire field of medicine that has revealed some breathtaking findings about its significance in human health. Indeed, getting quality sleep is a vital sign of well-being. Studies have convincingly proven that our sleep habits ultimately lord over everything about us—how much we eat, how fat we get, how strong our immune systems are, how creative and insightful we can be, how well we can cope with stress, how fast we can think, and how well we can remember things. Losing as few as one and a half hours that our body needs for just one night can reduce daytime alertness by about a third. Poor sleep habits equate with many scientifically proven consequences, among them: brain fog and memory loss, diabetes and obesity, cardiovascular disease, and depression.

---

hormone. But it actually helps control our entire twenty-four hour rhythm as well. Once released after the sun sets, it slows body function and lowers blood pressure and core body temperature so we're prepared to sleep.

Because so many hormones are related to sleep (some of which aren't released until you are asleep), getting adequate rest is a must. Ayurveda describes sleep as the "diet of the mind." It repairs and refreshes the mind and body on so many levels, it's no wonder we spend roughly a third of our life sleeping. Our pituitary gland, for instance, cannot begin to pump out growth hormone until we're asleep. A natural anti-aging substance, growth hormone does more than just stimulate cellular growth and proliferation; it affects almost every cell in the body, renewing its tissues and organs. It also rejuvenates the immune system and lowers the risk factors for heart attack, stroke, and osteoporosis. It even aids in our ability to maintain an ideal weight, helping us to burn fat for fuel.

Modern science has turned up some intriguing facts about the human body while studying its daily cycles. Turns out that our hands are hottest around 2:00 a.m. and we weigh the most at 7:00 p.m. Physical power and endurance is strongest in the early evening hours, and breathing problems tend to be more pronounced in the early morning hours. Coincidence? Not in the least. These biological mysteries are easily explained by understanding the body's relationship with the solar day.

Despite all the science about circadian rhythms we have today, Ayurveda has always recognized and appreciated nature's master cycles that mesh with human life, as well as the importance of sleep. And although we like to use clocks today, nature still abides by the ultimate composers of these underlying cycles: the sun and seasons. Our inner biological cycles that correspond with the outer cycles of nature are governed by the rising and setting sun (which changes throughout the year with the seasons) and are characterized by an integral relationship to the three doshas.

Every day, two primary cycles of change happen in the body, each containing a kapha, pitta, and vata phase. The first cycle occurs between sunrise and sunset, and the second between sunset and sunrise. The progression begins with kapha characteristics, followed by pitta and vata.

First Cycle (Day)

Kapha: 6:00 a.m.–10:00 a.m.

Pitta: 10:00 a.m.–2:00 p.m.

Vata: 2:00 p.m.–6:00 p.m.

Second Cycle (Night)

Kapha: 6:00 p.m.–10:00 p.m.

Pitta: 10:00 p.m.–2:00 a.m.

Vata: 2:00 a.m.–6:00 a.m.

You'll likely be sensitive during any period of the day or night that corresponds to your predominant dosha. This means you should be extra cautious about staying balanced during these times. Note that vata types tend to be light sleepers by nature. But that doesn't mean they need less sleep. Vata types need at least eight hours a night and might benefit from a nap during the day. Generally speaking, pitta types need fewer hours than vata types (six to eight), as they sleep soundly. Kapha types can spend too much time sleeping and would do well to stick with seven to eight hours nightly, while avoiding naps. Kapha types would also benefit from rising before or with the sun.

If you suffer from insomnia or fail to wake up feeling refreshed, excess vata is likely to blame. If ruminating or negative, worrisome thoughts keep you from falling asleep or if you wake up during the night in a sweat, excess pitta could be the culprit. And if you sleep like a rock, but it takes a great deal of effort to get out of bed in the morning (and you may also snore and have congestion), then excess kapha is probably the culprit.

Despite your individual dosha, here are some tips for a more restful night:

➤ Because the hours of sleep before midnight are the most rejuvenating of the night, it's critical to be in bed by 10:00 p.m. Every. Single. Night.

➤ Cultivate a peaceful, clean sleeping environment (no electronics in the bedroom).

➤ Avoid caffeine late in the day and be mindful of medications you take that can infringe on sleep.

➤ Take time before bed to unwind, disconnect from stimulating activities, and cue the body that it's time for rest. Try a warm bath, listening to soothing music, or light reading. Before lying down, try some deep-breathing exercises.

➤ Wear loose clothing to bed that's appropriate for the room temperature so you're not too hot or cold. Cooler bedrooms make for better sleep (between 65 and 70°F).

Bad dreams? Note that one of the best ways to spot a doshic imbalance is to notice a change in your dreams. If you start having intense, violent dreams, this may be a sign that pitta is surging for some reason. Pay attention to these clues and ask yourself what could be the cause. Sometimes it's just a passing speed bump in your life as you go through certain challenges or heightened periods of stress. And sometimes a string of restless nights can clue you in to a deeper imbalance. If you can become aware of the gathering storm early, you can intervene sooner and perhaps avert a serious derailment in your well-being.

Tip #2: Enjoy the Hot and Simple Sip: I cannot reiterate this simple tool enough: Drinking hot water throughout the day will stoke your digestive fire, improve digestion and the absorption of food, and help prevent the body from becoming clogged with ama. As noted earlier, avoid cold or carbonated drinks, especially with meals. Hot water also is a great aid in reducing food cravings between meals. The most purifying water is water that has been boiled for about ten minutes, as this precipitates out materials and reduces its heaviness (you will usually see a fine powder at the bottom of the pan). This also energizes the water.

Why does warm water work better than cold? In addition to warm water being closer to your body's temperature, which speeds digestion, think about the following: When you're cleaning a greasy pan, you don't use cold water to try and remove the sticky, slimy residue. You run the hot water and lather it up with soap. The same idea holds true on our insides: Warm water has a scraping and vasodilator effect—it will cleanse your insides and open up blood vessels to allow blood to flow more easily, which in turn aids digestion and other metabolic processes. Don't hesitate to add flavors to your water such as fresh lemon, mint, thyme, and ginger, as well as organic tea blends.

Tip #3: Make Time to Still Your Mind: Of all the pressures we deal with on a daily basis, I think it's safe to say most all of them share a relationship with time. We never seem to have enough of it. This is partly why we've forgotten how to live from dawn to dusk, as we follow an arbitrary clock rather than cues from nature about when we should be sleeping, eating, and engaged in activity. This creates a biological mismatch in us that can indeed have health implications. Taking a few minutes to still your mind each day is a way to dissolve stress, nurture creativity, and bring more balance to your relationship with nature and bodily rhythms. And one of the easiest, most effective ways to achieve this is through breath. Remember what I mentioned in Chapter 7: Breath is the single most important food. Through the process of breathing, we feed every cell of our body with prana, or the life force. Many different types of breathing techniques exist, some of which are as simple as sitting in silence with your eyes closed on the floor or on the front edge of a chair and focusing on a series of full, deep belly breaths that allow the diaphragm to perform its job effectively. This is called diaphragmatic breathing, and within minutes it can recharge the cells of the body with energy and infuse you with a greater awareness of how you breathe.

As we age, we tend to limit the movement of our diaphragm—the dome-shaped muscle located at the base of our rib cage between the stomach and lungs. The result is shallow or upper-chest breathing rather than authentic breathing during which the diaphragm contracts and pulls the bottom of the lungs downward, allowing you to bring in a full gulp of oxygen and then expel (exhale) carbon dioxide. Babies know how to breathe better than adults, so the next time you're looking for a model breather, check out a sleeping baby's rhythms and belly breaths. And then try it yourself. To make sure you're doing it correctly, it helps to place one hand on your abdomen so you can feel your stomach and lower rib cage move inward on the inhalation and expand outward on the exhalation. Keep your upper chest, neck, and shoulder muscles as relaxed as possible, but maintain a straight spine. Aim for a round of at least ten breaths per session.

One widely used breathing exercise you may encounter in a yoga class entails alternating which nostril inhales and exhales. This method is particularly good for balancing excess vata conditions of the mind. Ideally, do this on the floor while sitting in the cross-legged position or while sitting on the edge of a chair with your spine straight and your feet firmly pressed flat on the floor. Then, the steps for one cycle are as follows:

With your eyes shut, gently close your right nostril with the thumb of your right hand. Exhale through your left nostril and then slowly inhale as you feel your stomach expand outward. Gently close your left nostril with the ring and middle fingers of your right hand and slowly exhale through your right nostril. Keeping your left nostril closed, inhale through your right nostril. Close your right nostril with your thumb and again, exhale through your left nostril. That completes one full cycle. Aim to complete five cycles and work your way up to a daily practice that takes five minutes.

Meditation is a close cousin to deep-breathing exercises, and it's not just for Tibetan monks anymore. Although it requires nothing more in terms of "equipment" than a quiet space where you can sit comfortably (early morning and early evening are ideal times to meditate), it does demand some practice to master and should take about fifteen to twenty minutes. It's like exercise for the mind, and it often helps to learn the ropes to meditation through the help of a teacher or the use of a guided recording. Rarely are we truly "focused" today. We lead very scattered (and scatterbrained) lives, distracted by the frenzied competition that is our society. When was the last time you took a moment to sit and concentrate on just yourself without the dramas of life affecting you? No wonder meditation is so effective just by virtue of its permission to let you be calm, centered, and focused inward.

Plenty of sound research explains why meditation works. One of the most basic reasons is that it returns the brain to a more primitive state whereby we are less likely to hear the disruptive chatter from our usual judgmental and analytical selves. Before humans evolved into complex, critically thinking beings, our brains were a bit less complicated. We knew how to find food, water, and socialize to some degree, but we would have had a harder time with math, intricate future planning, and establishing sophisticated societies and cultures. But then we grew an outer neocortex, which added another layer to our brains so we could problem-solve better, build cities, and invent things like computers. With the yin of this more advanced human brain and a greater capacity to think came the yang of its disadvantage: We could be overly critical and super-judgmental to the point that we'd get in our own mental way. Which is where the practice of meditation comes into play.

The practice returns the human brain back to its pre-neocortex state, liberating us from our analytical, critical selves. In this state, you're aware of things but don't have any negativity. Researchers are finally beginning to understand how this happens and how it affects the aging process. In 2005 scientists at Massachusetts General Hospital published an imaging study showing that particular areas of the brain involved with attention and sensory processing are thicker in people who frequently meditate. This study also showed why meditation can promote a relaxed state. It appears that meditators can effectively shift their brain activity from one area to another, such as moving brain waves from a stress center to a calm one. Such physical shifting of brain activity to areas associated with relaxation explains why people who meditate are calmer and happier after their meditative session.

Scientists continue to study the link between the thickening of the cortex and better cognitive abilities (i.e., just because you have a thicker brain doesn't mean you're smarter). One thing is clear: The aging process naturally causes the cortex to thin out. And meditation can help you to maintain your cerebral thickness despite age. Meditation, as it were, is truly exercise for the brain. This puts a whole new spin on the idea of "use it or lose it." No doubt this boost helps us to make better decisions about our health and choose wisely when it comes to engaging in the kinds of habits that will contribute to ideal weight.

Although it helps to be trained in getting to a meditative state—a place where you're deeply relaxed, but still awake—it's actually easier than you think. You can start just by picking a word to repeat to yourself, like the familiar "*ommm.*" Other options include murmuring "breathe in" and "breathe out" to yourself, or counting your breaths from one to ten, then repeating. Close your eyes and focus on your word or count. Bring your attention back to the word or count if extraneous thoughts intrude. Continue this process for as long as you can without falling asleep. Set a timer for twenty minutes if you like, and when you're ready, slowly open your eyes.

We have a saying in Vedic culture: "word of mouth." It relates to the fact all of our problems are related to what we put in our mouth and what comes out of it, be it food or words. How true is that? If you've never given your mouth a rest by fasting for twelve hours and restraining from talking as much as possible, you might want to try it sometime. Give your mouth a rest, and reap numerous benefits.

Tip #4: Detox on the Equinox: Do the 21-day cycle of the diet (Phase 2) at least twice a year—once in the spring as you "wake up" to warmer months ahead (around March 20) and again around the fall equinox, when you prepare to "hibernate" for the colder months (around September 22). Alternatively, you can choose to do the 21-day cycle at the start of every new season (starting around the twenty-first or twenty-second day of September, December, March, and June, respectively). These are the times of year when most people are vulnerable to sickness as the weather shifts and allergies can strike as new irritants enter the air. The attention to diet will help you not only to cleanse the system, but to phase the body out of the previous season and ease into the new one.

Also consider classic Ayurvedic treatments, such as Panchakarma, twice a year. These programs entail massage, heat treatments, and internal cleansing therapies to prevent impurities from accumulating and to eliminate ama buildup in bodily tissues. A recent study published in *Alternative Therapies in Health and Medicine* documented a 50 percent reduction of the cancer-causing chemical PCB in the blood after five days of rejuvenation treatment, a specific program of Panchakarma.

Tip #5: Check in Routinely: Ask yourself how you're feeling on a regular basis and continue to correct yourself. This can be done daily, weekly, and monthly, depending on which goals you'd like to address and at what level you'd like to check in with yourself. You'd be surprised by what taking just three to five minutes during your day to assess how you feel and what you're thinking foremost about can do to your sense of well-being, peace of mind, and even your capacity to lose weight and set realistic goals for the future. Self-care begins with self-discovery. On a daily basis, for instance, it helps to ask yourself whether or not your body feels good and energetic in general. On a weekly or monthly basis, you may tune in to broader questions about yourself, such as whether or not you enjoy what you're doing professionally and if your work is satisfying. Aim to be mindful about everything going on in your life, from the joys of brushing your teeth to the trials and tribulations of maintaining enriching relationships (see Tip #12). Get into the habit of having insightful, inward conversations with yourself. Be mindful of what you're doing—every minute of the day. Try not to do anything in a zombie state of mind. Make sure that inner dialogue helps you to stay positive, upbeat, and present. Remember, self-reflection is an ongoing act that ultimately separates us from the physicality of the world and our more abstract personal constitution.

Committing your thoughts and ideas to paper can also make a huge difference. It affords you a record from which to look back in the future and simultaneously offers accountability. So few of us take the time anymore, during our hectic days serving and caring for others, to just turn the volume down on everyone and everything else. Following are some questions to help get you started if you don't know what to write about:

➤ What job or hobby would you like to try?
➤ What are the top three things on your bucket list (besides weight goals and typical to-dos)?
➤ What in life is causing you a great deal of stress and anxiety? How can you begin to remedy that, one step at a time?

➤ What are you most proud of? What gives you the strongest feelings of satisfaction and fulfillment?

You may find it helpful to keep multiple journals. In addition to one that records the more mundane, everyday tasks, you can maintain a journal that keeps track of your diet choices and physical activities, and another that stores your worries (a "worry journal" can be very handy for people who have a hard time getting to bed at night as stressful thoughts intrude). A worry journal by your bedside can act as a mental depository of your anxieties, and once you write them down, you close the book and tell yourself that you will deal with them tomorrow. You can also choose to keep a journal that keeps all of your positive notes and accomplishments. This is where you write down what went right during your day and what you are grateful for. Sometimes, on the worst of days, you can just be thankful that you got through it, and that you'll soon welcome a whole new day with promising thoughts and intentions.

Tip #6: Minimize Passive Entertainment While You Eat: So many of us eat while performing other tasks or being entertained by a television or computer. A calm and peaceful atmosphere promotes ideal digestion whereas one filled with diversion such as watching TV, reading, or engaging in heated discussions can compromise the entire digestive process. See if you can approach eating as a time to relax and recharge. Focus on the food, savoring its flavors and how it feels in your mouth. Sit down, close your eyes, be thankful for your food, and take small, conscious bites. Try holding your fork in the opposite, less dominant hand. This will automatically slow down the pace of your eating. Before you begin a meal, look down at your plate and ask: "Do I think this is good for me to eat at this time?"

Tip #7: Perform Regular Self-Oil Massage: As simple as it may sound, a few minutes of massage each morning is one of the most effective forms of preventive medicine. *Abhyanga*, "head-to-toe oil massage," is a staple in Ayurvedic practices. It nourishes the skin, calms the nervous system, removes impurities from the blood, and supports the inner tissues of the body. For vata types, sesame or almond oil is ideal, as these oils are rich and warming, to match your dominant dosha. For pitta types, a lighter, cooling oil like coconut or olive oil is ideal. And kapha types, who should perform self-oil massage a little less frequently, favor a lighter oil still, such as sunflower or grape-seed oil. Go for high-quality, organic, cold-pressed oils. Ideally, warm the oil first by immersing its container in a cup of hot water. Leave the oil on your skin for at least fifteen minutes (or up to thirty minutes) and follow with a hot shower or bath. Use circular strokes over your joints and abdomen, and up-and-down motions over your limbs.

If rubbing oil on your skin in the morning doesn't work with your routine, and you need to get showered and dressed quickly for work, then dry skin-brushing is an alternative (save the oil massage for an evening routine). You can purchase brushes specifically for this practice, which are made with natural bristles. Gently brush the skin before showering or bathing, as this will remove dead skin cells and help stimulate lymph flow.

Tip #8: Give Thanks Before Eating: This act isn't tied to any one faith or correct method. It's a way to honor the gift of food and the greater blessings of life. It's also a wonderful opportunity to downshift a few gears, slow down, bring a greater sense of awareness to the act of eating and your chosen foods, and get in synch with fellow diners and your environment, or just with yourself. During this time, the mind becomes quiet as your attention is turned toward the food and the blessing. This practice also brings a heightened appreciation for food and nourishment, which will foster healthy eating habits. You needn't try to dig up an old traditional prayer you heard as a kid. Just offer a simple blessing or thought of gratitude either out loud or in silence. You can use the same one before every meal, or make a new one up every time.

Tip #9: Make Lunch Your Biggest Meal of the Day (Eat Like a King During the Day, and a Pauper at Night): Many people "save up" their calories to feast on a banquet at dinner. But it's virtually impossible to make serious progress in your weight-loss goals if you continue to eat large evening meals. I cannot emphasize this point too much. Digestion is naturally weaker in the evening, and weaker still once you lie down to sleep. The body simply cannot take in and absorb large evening meals properly. If it tries to do so, much of that food will be digested poorly, setting you up for more ama, less agni, and greater challenges with weight.

Because digestion is strongest at midday, lunch is the time our body can best assimilate larger quantities of food. It should be the most important meal of the day, as you've already learned. After lunch, we still have many active hours to metabolize the food before winding down at night and going to bed.

Do your best to plan for and prepare your lunches, which should ideally be warm, cooked foods with a wide variety of tastes. I've given you plenty of warm lunch ideas on this diet. Remember, cold foods suppress digestion. Too many cold meals can result in indigestion, the accumulation of ama, and weight gain. Remember, too, that a hearty lunch will help you to feel less hungry in the evening, making it easier to stick to that all-important light evening meal.

Tip #10: Spice It Up! Add spices to your meals like fresh ginger, cumin, black pepper, turmeric, and fenugreek. For a list of must-have spices and herbs to have on hand in your kitchen, refer to page 98. Try to use as many of these as you can in your meal preparations. Many of them contain properties that will enhance your digestion and weight-loss goals.

Tip #11: Avoid Chronic Multitasking and Use Your Senses Sensibly:
Most of us try to do ten things at once today. And we inundate our
senses with incoming stimulators from various sources (think talking
on the phone while checking email and texting, while watching TV
or driving). But our brains don't like to multitask (believe it or not,
the brain effectively processes only one stream of information at a
time), and my guess is our hearts don't like it either. It's been estimated that more than a quarter of our workday is spent immersed
in information overload, much of which is inane data. This leads to
a lack of focus and smart thinking, not to mention the loss of a calm
body free of surges in stress and other weight-sabotaging hormones.
See if you can minimize the volume of multitasking you do each
day. Don't vigorously engage multiple senses at the same time that
requires your brain to constantly switch gears. This is why I recommend eating (sense of taste) in the absence of other activities. The
only exception I'll make: If watching TV while exercising motivates
you to keep a regular routine, then by all means do it. You can satisfy your body's need to move with your need to watch your favorite
show at the same time.

Remember, our senses continually shape our physical, mental,
emotional, and spiritual selves. We must use them wisely. In addition
to trying to do too many things at once, other ways we abuse our
senses involve surrounding ourselves with too much noise, watching violent programming on broadcast media, neglecting the body's
need for touch, and eating foods that aggravate our digestive systems. Now that you have greater tools for attaining balance in your
life, use them to stay attuned to your needs while liberating yourself
from any excesses that will clutter your body and mind.

Tip #12: Cultivate Healthy Relationships: How well do you relate
with other people? Is your marriage enriching or a source of hardship
and stress? Do you have a trusty set of friends? Do you like *yourself*?
You'd be surprised by how the nature of our health hinges on the na-

ture of our relationships. We are, after all, very social creatures. Relationships exist in all that we do and all that we are. In addition to relating with other human beings, you relate with the things around you—tangible objects, air to breathe, water to drink, food to eat, and, of course, nature. And you're continually relating to your own physical, mental, and spiritual well-being. Cultivating healthy relationships starts with establishing a healthy relationship with yourself first, which will then allow you to extend that inner love with others and all that surrounds you. Be honest with yourself; understand your intentions, your wishes, your aspirations, your desires, your needs, your strengths, and your weaknesses. Listen to your body and decipher between needless wants and true essentials. The more authentic you are with yourself, the better you can show up for others in your life and communicate with them openly. Of course, all this circles back to you and your capacity to make good decisions related to your health. The happier you are in your relationships, the easier it will be to make excellent decisions in all that you do.

I should also point out that it pays to be careful about faking health and happiness in your relationships. If you try to project happiness with others while suffering inside, this will work against you. I once treated a woman who came to me after her third failed marriage (an interesting tidbit: While happy marriages have been proven to increase longevity, unhappy marriages increase the chance of getting sick by 35 percent). She said that her marriages typically ended with a pattern of unhealthy eating habits that triggered colossal weight gain. She was hoping to avoid another cycle of weight gain now that she was going through another divorce. And the one area in her life that we addressed right away had nothing to do with food or her diet. It was her inner feelings of failure and unhappiness despite her feigned happiness toward friends and family. Once we changed that, we were able to then fix her relationship with food so that it became a source of nourishment and renewed life rather than a source of pain and illness.

Note: Even though we have more gadgets and apps now than ever to connect with others through phones and computers, we also have a higher number of people who are lonely and who harbor feelings of disconnectedness. It seems like the more connections we make on the surface, the more we lose out on opportunities to renew those much deeper, more rewarding connections in person. So to this end, see if you can nourish your relationships in authentic, intimate ways. Plan more time with the people who inspire, challenge, and de-stress you. And don't wait for the weekend! Regular quality time with the people dear to us can be incredibly therapeutic. When we reduce our isolation, we reduce our risk for emotional eating and illness, and we increase the quality of our lives.

Tip 13: Eat Less, Live Longer: It's been shown that people who win longevity contests simply eat less. They consume fewer calories overall than the general population. How is this achievable? In small bites, literally. To eat less, watch your portions (skip the second or third helping and push away from the table before you reach maximum fullness), save high-calorie foods for special occasions, avoid snacking, cook as much as you can instead of relying on prepared, packaged meals, shift the bulk of your eating to early in the day rather than later, and perhaps the best piece of advice in this department is to track your intake. Spend a day or two logging your meals and a rough estimate of your calorie consumption, as this can clue you in to just how much you're eating, and where you can likely cut corners.

Tip #14: Enjoy Nature's Beauty Frequently: So few of us spend time outdoors anymore. We live and work indoors often chained to electronics, meetings, and chores. But it's true that being outdoors and among plants and other living things can automatically enhance feelings of well-being while having a calming effect on your mind and nervous system. This is partly why going for walks and hikes, or sailing, or cycling—doing anything in the open air—can be so invigorating. So get out in nature as much as possible, whether you're a city slicker or a suburbanite. Find a park to take your daily walk in. Set up a chair in front of the window with the best view. Plan your workouts outside when the weather is agreeable. Walk barefoot on the earth for a few minutes every day, tuning in to the sensations under your feet. Take in the scenery and air along natural bodies of water. Enjoy the light and energy of the sun at dawn or dusk. Appreciate the "dark side" of nature, too, by gazing at the stars on a clear night. And don't forget to bring the outdoors inside. Decorate the room you spend the most time in with living plants. Philodendrons, for example, are hard to kill and will bring Mother Nature closer to you.

Tip #15: Be Consistent in Your Daily Routine: If the body didn't love consistency and predictability so much, then traveling across time zones and being out of synch with your usual routine wouldn't feel so awkward and uncomfortable. In fact, one of the surefire ways of reducing stress on your body and maintaining a balanced state of being (what traditional doctors would call "homeostasis") is to keep a steady daily routine year-round to the best of your ability, including weekends and holidays. I realize that social demands, unexpected events, and work obligations have us all breaking this rule once in a while, but see if in the least you can automate the two biggest areas in your life that will have a huge impact in your body's balancing act: when you eat and sleep. If you can regulate just these two habits in your life, you will notice a difference in how you feel. It may also help you to regulate your exercise routine as well, which will also help you to stick to a routine.

Tip #16: Seek Variety in Life's Bigger Picture: Remember how exciting that first day of kindergarten or first grade was? It's thrilling to enter a new environment, meet new people, be exposed to fresh ideas, and learn something different. As adults we have enough to keep up with in our daily obligations, so we rarely give ourselves permission to act like a schoolgirl or -boy again, but doing so can actually have some surprising benefits. In addition to expanding your horizons, trying something out of your box can give you the feeling that you're on vacation, that you're allowed to goof off and replenish the kid in you again who's unencumbered by the banalities of everyday life.

Think about your current hobbies or one you'd like to try and see if you can find a club, group, or class nearby in which to participate. This can be any number of things, including a cooking class, a writing class, a pottery workshop, a photo club, or a book club. And if you can't find anything attuned to your interests, then start your own group and invite your friends.

To this end, don't forget to include volunteerism in your dose of variety. Though the media likes to focus on how giving back is the practical way in which each one of us can have an impact in the world and effect global change, I like to think about what it gives the person who is doing the giving back: a chance to forge new friendships and do something different. We know that there's a connection between volunteer work and longevity; it goes without saying that joyful people live longer. Case in point: Men who volunteer once a week have half the death rate of those who don't. This is probably true for women as well. The act of volunteering satisfies so many health-promoting aspects of our lives, from feeding our deep-seated wish to give back to making us feel connected, loved, and needed. All of this, in turn, nourishes our soul and supports a healthy physiology through feel-good body chemistry. Just be sure that whatever you do, you engage in activities that help you feel lighter and happier. Avoid anything that comes with heavy emotions that will literally weigh you down.

Tip #17: Free Yourself from Addictions: Clearly, it's beyond the scope of this book to teach you how to end your addictions that take away from your health and quality of life. Whether it's a dependency on drugs, nicotine, or alcohol, or just a habit of overeating and bingeing on ice cream every night, addiction prevents us from achieving balance and living an authentic life. Do what you can to work toward addressing your addictions, even if that means entering a traditional treatment program or consulting a professional. The Hot Belly Diet can enhance any additional efforts you employ to deal with your addictions. In fact, many of the ideas I've already presented, such as learning to meditate, retooling your diet, daily oil massage, and engaging in regular exercise will go a long way to help you treat your addictions regardless of what else you do. These practices are automatically calming to the nervous system—the very system that's often in charge of fueling and feeding your addictions. One of the most important things to keep in mind as you come to grips with an addiction is that it needn't define your life, and that you haven't "ruined everything." The negativity that comes with an addiction, including the pain that it often inflicts on loved ones, is not you. It's the result of physical and mental ama that's been allowed to accumulate over time. Just be sure to avoid programs that use confrontational tactics, which feed feelings of guilt, shame, blame, and remorse. Ayurveda teaches the opposite: When an addict finds a source of balance, pleasure, and satisfaction outside of the object of addiction (e.g., cigarettes, alcohol, food), the urge to remain an addict subsides. So the goal is to expose the addict to new sources of satisfaction that distract him or her from the addiction, which is exactly what an Ayurvedic approach to life can help one achieve.

Tip #18: Be Honest with Yourself When You Need to Take a Time-Out: It's all too common these days for us to push through feelings of illness and pain and the urge to take a break to just relax. Some of us don't even take advantage of (paid) vacation time anymore. But it's essential that we let our body gather strength and energy routinely during planned downtimes rather than let all that stress build up. Although it sounds cliché to say "relax" because it will "reduce stress," it's all the more important today because we seem to value busy-ness so much. Stress will always be a part of our life; the key is to keep certain sources of unnecessary stress at bay so they don't affect us like a charging bull. Easier said than done, but here are some things to think about: Can you set a time each day after which you turn off your cell phone and don't respond to nonemergency calls, emails, text messages, and so on? Can you treat yourself once a month or as often as feasible to a massage or other therapeutic treatment of your choice? Can you pick one single habit you want to change and make a commitment to making that happen? It can be an ambitious goal like quitting smoking or a small one like reducing your consumption of fast food or avoiding late-night eating.

Tip #19: Pursue Your Passions and Live to the Fullest of Your Unique Self: Not all of us can say we are 100 percent satisfied with our current jobs. But as the old saying goes, "If you love your job, you don't have to work for a single day in your life." I marvel with sadness at the fact a great majority of us are not happy in our work. Some of us walk around with a keen sense of who we are and what we want to become in life, whereas others feel less certain and continually struggle to find those answers. No matter where you are in your own emotional journey, it helps to examine your attitude and perspectives.

While it can take time, patience, and trial and error to find and flourish in a career that's deeply fulfilling and enriching, that doesn't mean you can't find a certain level of enjoyment and gratification in whatever job helps you meet your obligations now. You will continue to explore opportunities in the hopes of finding and establishing yourself in the ideal work scenario. After all, in any job there's bound to be periods of frustration, high stress, and maybe anguish. Even people who are lucky to have already found their dream job experience challenges that require them to refocus or test a new and unplanned path. Taking stock of your feelings about your work-life is critical to your personal weight-loss plan. Your emotional health is a big piece of the diet puzzle, constituting that third dimension to overall wellness. We spend the majority of our days working, so it's vital that those long days are contributing to our mental and physical health—not taking away. This is possible when we strive to align our goals and values with our talents and passions in a job that supports our livelihood, and allows us to feel appreciated and needed in the world at large. And don't forget to make room for fun and laugher in whatever job you pursue. The act of laughter itself will make you feel lighter and heighten your sense of awareness. A belly full of laughs is a hot belly indeed.

Tip #20: Embrace an Active Sex Life: If sexual intimacy were not a magnificent source of pleasure, then it probably wouldn't have such a positive impact on our health. The science is well documented: Having a strong sexual appetite and the ability to perform sex is indicative of overall health, longevity, and tissue function. It plays into our immunity, mental wellness, and our ojas, our essential life energy. It also helps us connect with another human being in a special kind of relationship that nourishes us on so many levels. A healthy relationship with sex, including its emotional component, is important. Sex should not be misused or lead to an imbalance of any sort.

Ayurveda believes that nighttime is the ideal time for sex, rather than the morning and daytime. It also encourages more sex during the colder months of the year rather than during the hotter months, when there's a greater loss of energy and fluids from the body. Few books on health today dare to talk about sex, which is often relegated to books dedicated solely to the subject. But I bring this up because I want you to keep in mind the value that an active sex life brings to your life, and your ability to achieve and maintain an ideal weight. Just as we need water, food, and oxygen to live, so do we need to practice one of the greatest creative forces through which we can express and share our love.

Tip #21: Love and Be Loved: I once read somewhere that people who work with dying individuals in hospice-care facilities often hear the same questions from those going through the process of dying: Am I loved? And did I love well? They are at a point in their life when all the trivial sources of stress are gone and all that's left to ponder is the extent and capacity of their love. Love is, after all, the ultimate medicine, antidote, cure, and treatment. It's everything. When you are loved and you love well, every cell in your body is allowed to work at its maximum capacity. The ideas and strategies in this book will help you to let love inside and give love out, and as you experience more love in your life, you will automatically develop a greater understanding of yourself and the world at large. If love is the single most important ingredient to health and wellness, then I know of no better way of staying on the path of continual healing than to love as much as you can.

CHAPTER 10

Odds and Ends in Classic Q&A

You can live to be a hundred if you give up all the things that you want to live to be a hundred.

—WOODY ALLEN

Perhaps Woody Allen stated it best when he implied that longevity does hinge a bit on things we may not want to do (and that dovetails one of Mark Twain's famous remarks: "The only way to keep your health is to eat what you don't want, drink what you don't like, and do what you'd rather not"). Indeed, a healthy life must include some restraint and self-control. There's plenty of room for splurges and liberties of all kinds, but those must be tempered with the healing powers of judicious limitations. This, after all, is the essence of honoring and loving the human body for both its needs and wants.

To help you further solidify the concepts of this book and manage any challenges you may have now or going forward, let me share the answers to the top questions I get from people who are embarking on my program or who have completed it. These have the effect of doing two things: (1) reiterating key takeaways from the book and (2) equipping you with some troubleshooting advice if you don't feel like you've achieved what you want yet out of the program. Don't forget to also visit me at www.hotbellydiet.com for more up-to-date information, resources, and opportunities to ask questions and share your experience with other fellow dieters in your journey.

Q. What if I get hungry in between meals?

A. Remember, one of the most important strategies of the Hot Belly Diet is to avoid snacking so your body can experience the rewards of mild intermittent fasting. So first try taking some sips of warm water, and getting up and moving around (go outside for some fresh air). And if you still cannot get rid of your hunger pang, then have a piece of whole, low-sugar fruit (choose from the list on page 99).

Q. I've gotten headaches while on the diet. What can I do to minimize them? Why are they stronger than normal?

A. This is a common response to the diet, especially if you're someone who was eating poorly (i.e., lots of processed foods) before. Because the diet has a detoxifying effect on the body, you feel this effect with a headache. It's actually a good sign that the diet is working. Part of the pain can be from withdrawing from caffeine, too. Don't panic: The headaches will not continue. By the second half of the Accelerate Phase, not only will your headaches wane, but you'll be much less likely to experience them in the future than before you even started the diet. So stay strong and help alleviate those headaches by hydrating as much as possible. Be sure to keep drinking warm water or herbal teas throughout the day. If you were used to drinking coffee prior to commencing the diet, then be sure to at least prepare green tea for your morning fix, as this contains some caffeine to avert that withdrawal.

Q. I'm not sleeping well due to the light dinner. What can I do?

A. Admittedly, it takes time to get used to the lighter supper, especially if you were accustomed to making dinner your biggest meal. Rather than heading to the refrigerator, though, try drinking some chamomile tea or other warm herbal tea before bed. If you find yourself lying there in bed unable to go to sleep, mentally center your mind and focus on your breathing. Make sure your inner-self talk remains calm and fixated on the health benefits that are happening at that moment. Don't think about hunger or the urge to go to the kitchen. This mental wrestling and "insomnia" will go away the longer you stay the course.

Q. Where can I buy the khichadi rather than having to prepare it myself from scratch?

A. Go to my website at www.hotbellydiet.com for resources.

Q. If I take castor oil and nothing happens, what do I do? How long do I wait to repeat?

A. As I mentioned earlier, some people don't respond to the oil cleanse within three to four hours. Be patient if nothing happens that first day. If, on the other hand, you're still waiting on the second day's afternoon to pay a visit to the bathroom for a strong bowel movement, then repeat the protocol. Most people will respond rather quickly to that first dose. Just be sure to avoid doubling the dose within twenty-four hours, as you may find yourself uncomfortable.

Q. Am I getting enough protein and fiber while on the diet?

A. Yes and yes. People have a tendency to think they need a lot more protein than they really do (and it doesn't help that food products today reiterate false ideas about our protein needs). Not only does the Hot Belly Diet deliver plenty of high-quality protein to the body, but it also contains an abundance of natural fiber as found in the fresh vegetables, whole grains, and fruits. If you feel constipated, then try a high-quality fiber supplement from psyllium husk. And if you truly feel like you're not getting enough protein, perhaps because you're a very active individual, then make sure you choose high-protein breakfasts and lunches. You can do this by having a Superfood Smoothie (page 233) for breakfast with a hard-boiled egg and including lean protein in the form of fish, turkey, chicken, or tofu with your lunch.

Q. Can I add some other vegetables apart from what you've listed?

A. Of course, but try to stick to my lists as much as possible during the Accelerate Phase. You can branch out and add more variety during the Transform Phase by adding other leafy greens available to you. Just be careful about starchy, sugary vegetables.

Q. I don't feel like the weight is coming off fast enough. What could be wrong?

A. Nothing is wrong if you're following the diet carefully. You might not see results on the scale right away, but your body is certainly undergoing lots of positive changes at the cellular, hormonal, and molecular levels. It's also adjusting to your new way of eating (and hopefully moving!). Soon enough, you'll be *feeling* different in your clothes, and this can happen before you see the scale tick downward. Be patient. By the second and third weeks, you should see results.

Q. What do I do with my Western drugs? Do I keep taking my blood-pressure and cholesterol-lowering medications, for example?

A. Yes, continue with your prescribed medications as you've been taking them. Should you have any concerns, ask your doctor. With the exception of pregnancy and breast-feeding women (see next question), this diet is compatible with any condition.

Q. I'm pregnant/breast-feeding. Can I do the program?

A. You are the one exception. It's best for you to wait until you're not pregnant and are done breast-feeding before embarking on this diet. Nutritional needs during this time in a woman's life are very different and unique. Even though the Hot Belly Diet is a nutritionally balanced, complete program, it's not a good idea to aim to lose weight under these circumstances without a doctor's approval and monitoring. So speak with the physician who is caring for you while pregnant first.

Q. I've always been an active workout person. Can I keep up my routine when I start this diet?

A. Even if you're an avid exerciser (and for that you get an extra star), I advise that you avoid excessively strenuous workouts during the Accelerate Phase, while your body is readjusting to a new metabolic rhythm. You can then return to your favorite exercise during the Transform Phase. Note that people who exercise tend to need more calories than sedentary people, since they are burning more energy and typically have faster metabolisms as a result. So as you ease back into your regular exercise routine, especially if it's rigorous, be mindful of your body's caloric needs. Add more by choosing more vegetables and high-quality lean proteins. Avoid the cheap, nutrient-poor calories in sugary, processed foods, and energy bars and drinks.

Q. Can I eat in a restaurant for lunch?

A. Although it helps to avoid restaurants as much as possible during the Accelerate Phase, if you get stuck having to eat in a restaurant, order fresh salads with steamed vegetables and good-quality organic animal protein (preferably baked without heavy sauces or coatings). And don't load down your salads with cheese and creamy dressings. Try a drizzle of olive oil vinaigrette and a squeeze of lemon.

Q. I'm more snappy and irritable since starting the diet. Why?

A. This is normal as your body adjusts and goes through a slight withdrawal from the processed, packaged (or otherwise low-quality) foods you may have been eating before. Just relax. Go out for a walk when your mood takes a dip. Talk to a friend or engage in an activity that you find enjoyable and that reliably elevates your mood. Most important, don't let this emotion take you to the refrigerator. This moodiness goes away toward the end of the second phase.

Q. I have only five pounds to lose. Can I do just half of the program? Fifteen days instead of thirty?

A. No matter how much or how little you want to lose, I recommend staying on the diet for its full duration so you can completely train your body to effortlessly gravitate toward this way of eating for life. Remember, this isn't just about losing weight, and it takes about a month to form a new, reliable habit. One thing to keep in mind, however: If you find yourself losing weight too quickly and you start to go past your target, then increase the quantity of the khichadi at your lunch or dinner and add more cleansing vegetables and high-quality lean protein.

Q. Is this diet safe for anyone regardless of age?

A. Indeed, this protocol has been used for millennia safely among millions. I've seen numerous benefits among people in my practice regardless of age. The end game isn't just about losing weight. Many things will vanish, from daily nuisances like headaches and skin conditions to serious challenges like insulin resistance and risk for life-threatening illnesses. Even if you have a chronic condition today, this diet can work for you.

Q. How many bowel movements should I have a day?

A. Everyone will be different in this department, but most should have at least one healthy bowel movement per day.

Q. I've already done the Hot Belly Diet and achieved the results I wanted. But if I don't want to follow the entire 30-day protocol to the T in the future, what can I do to renew and rejuvenate my body quickly?

A. Whenever you feel like your body needs a break and could use a refresher, I can't think of a better strategy than to fast. It's a panacea of sorts. As I noted earlier, fasting is an excellent way to stoke that agni fire and burn away ama from the body. For centuries, various cultures have endorsed fasting as a means to reboot the body from a physical, mental, emotional, and spiritual standpoint. And we know from modern science that fasting does have its metabolic and even brain-enhancing benefits. Although we tend to think of negative effects when we deprive the body of calories, let alone cause it to go into "starvation mode," studies now show that calorie restriction can have tremendously positive effects on the body, turning on pathways that boost brain function (and even the birth of new brain cells), activating the body's internal antioxidant network, and heightening the body's immune system (when calories are reduced in the diets of laboratory animals, for example, not only do they live longer, but they also become remarkably resistant to the development of several cancers). Fasting not only turns on health-promoting genetic machinery, but also powers up the body's internal healing methods, leading to enhanced detoxification and a reduction of inflammation. Simply put, fasting enhances energy production and paves the way for better physiological function and mental clarity.

Ayurveda encourages short-term, intermittent fasting throughout the year to clear out digestive clutter, improve mental clarity, and preserve overall health. This can be done in combination with the Hot Belly Diet protocol (remember, you could swap the castor oil cleanse for a day of fasting during which you consume only liquids in the form of warm water, hot teas, and brothy soups; it's an excellent way to set the foundation for and speed up your body's shift to burning fat for fuel and producing biochemicals that have astonishing pro-health effects on the body). Or you can set aside a day or so on a monthly or seasonal basis for fasting. I recommend that you at least try to plan for a complete restriction of solid food for twenty-four to seventy-two hours at regular intervals two to four times annually (see #3 on page 232). If this is too difficult to do, then aim for a fast that includes just fruits, vegetables, and juices (#2 below).

Although the old conventional wisdom said that fasting lowers the metabolism and forces the body to hold on to fat in a so-called starvation mode, the new science proves that fasting provides the body with benefits that can accelerate and enhance weight loss, not to mention that it improves general health on many levels.

The exact type of fast you choose and for how long will depend on your individual needs and personal constitution, including your digestive strength, level of ama, and overall vitality. Any ongoing health challenges should be taken into consideration as well. If you take any medications, continue to take them (if you take diabetes medications, please consult your physician first; I recommend that you speak with your doctor if you have any chronic conditions before commencing a fasting protocol).

Generally speaking, the four different fasting protocols—from least to most vigorous—entail the following:

1. Consuming light, easily digestible foods only, such as khichadi, soupy broths, and warm herbal teas.
2. Eating fruits, vegetables, or juices only.
3. Avoiding solid foods and drinking water or herbal teas.
4. Avoiding both food and water (limit to twenty-four hours).

Fasting should not feel like drudgery. Nor should it be done during a stressful time period or when you cannot stick to the fast easily due to other obligations. Signs of an effective fast include lightness in the body, clarity in the mind, and increased energy. Your bowel movements will become more regular, and you'll be free of excess gas and bloating. You'll have a clean tongue and fresh breath. And when you're ready to resume your usual dietary regimen after the fast, do so gradually and slowly, working your way back to solid meals again. Avoid overeating once the fast is over, and choose foods that won't be difficult to digest.

Appendix A: The Hot Belly Diet Recipes

SUPERFOOD SMOOTHIE

Serves 1

⅔ cup unsweetened almond milk or rice milk (no soy milk)

⅔ cup water

2 scoops protein powder in the form of whey isolate, hemp seed protein powder, or brown rice protein powder

1 tablespoon whole flaxseed, shelled hemp seeds, or raw sunflower seeds, and a small handful of blueberries, raspberries, or blackberries

Pinch of cinnamon, pinch of nutmeg, and/or pinch of cardamom powder (choose two of these three)

Mix all the ingredients in a blender.

Variation: For added sweetness, add 1 teaspoon of unheated raw honey or Stevia. Those who don't want to use almond or rice milk can opt for ¼ cup yogurt (1% fat Greek-style yogurt) or ¼ cup kefir and 1 cup water instead.

Note: Play with different berries, types of milk, flavors of protein (a list of brands to look for can be found at www.hotbellydiet.com; the product will include the scoop for measuring), and seeds on a daily basis.

COCONUT-CUCUMBER SMOOTHIE

Serves 1

½ small cucumber

½ cup unsweetened organic coconut milk

½ cup unsweetened organic rice milk

1½ cups chopped watercress

½ teaspoon maple syrup

Juice the cucumber in a juicer.

Pour the cucumber juice into a blender and add the remaining ingredients. Blend until smooth.

Pour the smoothie into a chilled glass and drink.

MIDDAY KHICHADI

Serves 1

¼ cup basmati rice or buckwheat (use organic)

½ cup split mung beans (use organic)

2½ cups water

2 teaspoons olive oil

1½ teaspoons curry powder

Salt

3 to 4 stems and leaves of fresh cilantro, finely chopped

1 cup finely chopped cleansing vegetables (see page 98)

1 tablespoon raw, unsalted seeds of your choice (see options, page 98)

2 tablespoons chopped raw nuts of your choice (see options, page 98)

Rinse the rice and beans. In a medium pot, combine the water, beans, and rice and bring to a boil. Reduce the heat to a low boil and continue cooking for 20 to 30 minutes. Add the oil, curry powder, and salt while cooking. Stir well in between.

At the end, add the cilantro, vegetables, seeds, and nuts. Stir well and serve hot.

SUPPERTIME KHICHADI

Serves 2 to 3

Repeat the Midday Khichadi recipe (page 234), but replace the cleansing vegetables (see page 98) with your choice of 1 cup finely chopped leafy greens: lettuce, spinach, kale, chard, collard greens, arugula, turnip greens, leeks, and cilantro. Also, replace the rice or buckwheat with ¼ cup quinoa, and skip the nuts.

GOURMET KHICHADI

Serves 4 to 6

2½ cups water

¼ cup split yellow mung beans

½ cup white basmati rice, rinsed

1 cup chopped or grated carrots

1 cup chopped parsnips

1 tablespoon chopped fresh ginger

3 tablespoons ghee

1 teaspoon mustard seeds

½ cup chopped onion

½ teaspoon coriander powder

½ teaspoon cumin powder

½ teaspoon turmeric powder

1 dried chili pepper, chopped or torn

½ teaspoon freshly ground black pepper

½ teaspoon rock salt

Freshly squeezed juice of ½ lemon or lime

3 to 5 fresh basil leaves (or fresh cilantro leaves), chopped

Combine the water, mung beans, rice, carrots, parsnips, and ginger in a stockpot, cover, bring to a boil, and then reduce the heat to a simmer.

Heat the ghee in a second pan and then add the mustard seeds; cook until the seeds begin to pop. Add the onion, coriander, cumin, turmeric, chili pepper, and black pepper and fry until the onion is slightly browned. Then combine everything in the second pan. Add the rock salt, lemon juice, and basil.

YOGURT PARFAIT WITH LOW-FAT GRANOLA

Serves 1

1 cup low-fat, low-sugar
   vanilla or plain yogurt

½ cup organic granola

½ cup fresh berries

In a large glass, layer ½ cup of the yogurt, ¼ cup of the granola, and ¼ cup of the berries. Repeat the layers.

CLASSIC SWEET LASSI

Serves 1

½ cup organic plain yogurt

1½ cups water

2 teaspoons raw honey or
   turbinado sugar

¼ teaspoon cardamom

Mix all the ingredients in a blender until smooth. Serve in chilled glasses.

SALTY (DIGESTIVE) LASSI

Serves 1

½ cup organic plain yogurt

1½ cups water

½ teaspoon cumin seeds

¼ teaspoon salt

3 to 4 fresh leaves of mint, or
   1 to 2 stems of cilantro

Mix all the ingredients in a blender until smooth. Serve in chilled glasses.

WILD RICE SALAD WITH FENNEL

Serves 2

¾ cup dried wild rice, soaked
    for ½ hour, rinsed and
    drained, then cooked for
    ½ hour or until done

1 green apple, peeled,
    cored, and diced

1 fennel bulb, diced

Roasted walnuts (1 handful
    or more to taste)

Handful of currants soaked
    in cranberry juice (or
    freshly squeezed juice
    of 1 blood orange)

Dressing:

Juice of 1 lemon

1 to 2 tablespoons olive oil

1 tablespoon balsamic vinegar

¼ teaspoon salt

2 to 4 tablespoons finely
    chopped fresh fennel grass

1 teaspoon crushed fennel seeds

1½ cups finely chopped
    fresh Italian parsley

Combine all the ingredients and serve immediately.

KALE AND MANDARIN SALAD

Serves 4

Bunch of kale, chopped
    into bite-size pieces

2 mandarins, segmented

1 carrot, shredded

¼ cup cranberries

½ cucumber, peeled and
    thinly sliced

1 medium tomato, diced

1 tablespoon toasted
    sunflower seeds

2 tablespoons coconut flakes

Salt

2 tablespoons olive oil

Combine all the ingredients, toss, and serve.

PERSIMMON SALAD WITH FENNEL

Serves 4

2 small Fuyu persimmons

1 small to medium fennel bulb

¾ head frisée lettuce

4 to 5 tablespoons olive oil

2 tablespoons balsamic vinegar

Salt and freshly ground
    black pepper

⅓ cup walnut pieces

Slice the persimmons thinly after cored, seeded, and halved. Place in a salad bowl.

Slice the fennel and add to the bowl.

Break the frisée into bite-size pieces and add to the bowl.

Whisk the oil, vinegar, salt, and pepper in another bowl, then add the walnuts. Drizzle the desired amount of dressing on the salad and toss.

CITRUSY KALE SALAD WITH BLUEBERRIES AND PUMPKIN SEEDS

Serves 2

Bunch of curly kale

2 tablespoons olive oil

¾ teaspoon sea salt plus more to taste

Zest and juice of 1 lemon

Zest and juice of 1 orange

1 teaspoon honey

Freshly ground black pepper

½ ripe avocado, cubed

1 cup fresh blueberries

2 tablespoons toasted or raw pumpkin seeds

Remove the kale leaves from the stem and chop into bite-size pieces (or tear using your hands).

Place the kale in a large bowl and drizzle 1 tablespoon of the oil and the salt onto the leaves, massaging with your hands. Do this for a few minutes, thoroughly massaging the oil into the leaves.

Set aside (the leaves should begin to wilt).

Whisk the lemon and orange juice and zest, the remaining 1 tablespoon oil, and the honey. Season with salt and pepper to taste. Pour the dressing over the kale leaves.

Add the avocado, blueberries, and pumpkin seeds and toss. Serve.

Note: Instead of blueberries and pumpkin seeds try any of the following:

Blackberries and walnuts

Sliced strawberries and pecans

Raspberries and sliced almonds

TUSCAN KALE

Serves 6 to 8

2 tablespoons dried currants

7 tablespoons white balsamic vinegar

1 tablespoon honey

1 tablespoon extra-virgin olive oil

1 teaspoon salt plus more to taste

2 bunches of Tuscan kale (about 1 pound), ribs and stems removed, leaves thinly sliced crosswise

2 tablespoons pine nuts, lightly toasted

Salt and freshly ground black pepper

Parmesan cheese shavings

Place the currants in a small bowl; add 5 tablespoons of the vinegar. Let soak overnight. Drain the currants.

Whisk the remaining 2 tablespoons vinegar, honey, oil, and salt in a large bowl.

Add the kale, currants, and pine nuts; toss to coat. Let marinate for 20 minutes at room temperature, tossing occasionally.

Season with salt and pepper. Sprinkle Parmesan over the salad and serve.

EDAMAME-QUINOA SALAD

Serves 4

Salad:

1 cup quinoa, rinsed

½ teaspoon salt

1 cup shelled edamame

1½ cups halved cherry or grape tomatoes

1 cup finely chopped red cabbage

1 cup diced cucumber

Dressing:

½ cup olive oil

¼ cup freshly squeezed lemon juice

2 tablespoons maple syrup

1 tablespoon Dijon mustard

1 teaspoon salt

To make the salad, bring the quinoa, salt, and 1½ cups of water to a boil in a saucepan. Reduce the heat to medium-low, cover, and simmer for 20 minutes, or until the water is absorbed. Set aside, covered, for 10 minutes.

Bring 2 cups of water to a boil in a separate saucepan. Add the edamame and cook for 1 minute. Drain and rinse under cold water. Drain again. Stir the edamame, tomatoes, cabbage, cucumber, and quinoa in a bowl.

To make the dressing. Mix all the ingredients in a blender until smooth. Stir into the salad.

KALE TABBOULEH

Serves 4

⅔ cup fine bulgur

3 tablespoons freshly squeezed lemon juice

1 shallot, finely chopped

2 teaspoons ground cumin

1¼ teaspoons fine sea salt plus more as needed

½ cup extra-virgin olive oil plus more as needed

1 bunch of kale, stems removed, leaves finely chopped (about 5 cups)

2 large ripe tomatoes, diced (about 2 cups)

½ cup torn mint leaves

½ cup diced radishes

Salt and freshly ground black pepper

Cook the bulgur according to the package directions. Let cool.

In a small bowl, whisk the lemon juice, shallot, cumin, and salt. Whisk in the olive oil.

In a large bowl, toss the bulgur, kale, tomatoes, mint, and radishes. Toss in the dressing. Season with salt and black pepper, and drizzle with additional oil, if desired.

BUTTERNUT SQUASH AND SPINACH CURRY

Serves 6

2 tablespoons vegetable oil

1 large onion, chopped

1 medium butternut squash
(about 2¾ pounds), peeled
and cut into ¾-inch cubes

2 garlic cloves, crushed

2 to 3 tablespoons curry paste

1 (14-ounce) can diced tomatoes

1½ cups vegetable or chicken
broth plus more as needed

1 (8-ounce) bag fresh baby
spinach, rinsed

Salt and freshly ground
black pepper

Low-fat yogurt (optional)

Heat the oil in a large deep pan, add the onion, and cook for 2 to 3 minutes. Add the butternut squash, garlic, and curry paste and cook for 2 to 3 minutes more.

Add the tomatoes and broth. Bring to a boil, then reduce the heat, cover, and simmer for 15 minutes, stirring occasionally. Remove the lid and simmer for 10 minutes. Add extra broth or water if necessary.

Stir in the spinach, cover, and cook for 1 to 2 minutes, until wilted. Season to taste with salt and pepper, and spoon into serving bowls, topping with low-fat yogurt, if desired.

STRAWBERRY, ALMOND, AND ARUGULA SALAD

Serves 2

½ cup almonds

2 tablespoons white wine vinegar

1 teaspoon cumin seeds

1 teaspoon poppy seeds

1 teaspoon honey

½ cup olive oil

Kosher salt

Freshly ground black pepper

3 cups baby arugula or watercress,
thick stems trimmed

8 ounces fresh strawberries, halved or quartered if large (about 2 cups)	1 ounce Parmesan cheese, shaved

Preheat the oven to 350°F. Spread the almonds on a small rimmed baking sheet and toast, tossing occasionally, until golden brown, 8 to 10 minutes. Let cool.

Whisk the vinegar, cumin seeds, poppy seeds, and honey in a large bowl. Whisk in the oil; season with salt and pepper.

Add the arugula, strawberries, and almonds to the vinaigrette; toss to coat. Top with the Parmesan.

POTATO-RASPBERRY SALAD*

Serves 6

4 large red potatoes	½ teaspoon honey
1 cup fresh raspberries	1 tablespoon finely chopped fresh sage
4 cups mixed leafy greens, such as arugula and baby spinach	1 tablespoon sesame seeds
½ cup snap peas	¼ teaspoon sea salt
½ large red onion, thinly sliced	¼ teaspoon crushed red pepper
1 tablespoon coconut oil, melted	¼ teaspoon freshly ground black pepper

Bring a large pot of lightly salted water to a boil over medium heat; add the potatoes and cook for about 20 minutes, or until tender. Remove from the heat; drain and run under cool water for 1 minute. Dice the potatoes and place in a large bowl.

Add the remaining ingredients and toss to combine.

Transfer to serving bowls; serve warm.

HONEY QUINOA*

Serves 4

1½ cups quinoa

1 tablespoon honey

⅓ cup finely chopped fresh cilantro

⅓ cup honey-roasted peanuts

Juice of 1 orange

2 teaspoons fresh orange zest

2 scallions, thinly sliced

¼ teaspoon sea salt

¼ teaspoon freshly ground black pepper

Cook the quinoa according to the package directions. Remove from the heat and immediately transfer to a large bowl. Add the honey; gently toss to combine. Set aside, covered, for 10 minutes to allow the honey to absorb.

Combine the remaining ingredients and add to the bowl.

Transfer to serving bowls. Serve warm or chilled.

LEMON SQUASH SALAD*

Serves 4

1 medium yellow squash, cut into ½-inch pieces

2 cups cooked teff (gluten-free grain)

1 cup steamed baby spinach

2 scallions, thinly sliced

½ medium red onion, thinly sliced

3 tablespoons fresh lemon juice

1 teaspoon balsamic vinegar

1 tablespoon lemon zest

2 tablespoons extra-virgin olive oil

2 teaspoons ground chia seeds

½ teaspoon sea salt

¼ teaspoon freshly ground black pepper

1 large head Bibb lettuce

1 tablespoon finely chopped fresh cilantro for garnish

In a large bowl, combine the squash, teff, spinach, scallions, and onion.

To make the dressing, whisk the lemon juice, vinegar, lemon zest, oil, chia seeds, sea salt, and pepper in a separate small bowl.

Pour the dressing over the squash mixture; gently toss to combine.

Tear apart pieces of the Bibb lettuce and place in serving dishes. Divide the teff mixture on top. Garnish with the fresh cilantro.

WATERMELON SALAD*

Serves 4

2 cups ½-inch chunks yellow watermelon

2 cups ½-inch chunks pink watermelon

1 cup fresh blueberries

6 fresh strawberries, quartered

3 cups packed baby mixed greens

2 teaspoons fresh lemon zest

2 tablespoons sesame seeds

1 teaspoon Dijon mustard

2 tablespoons apple cider vinegar

2 tablespoons flaxseed oil

½ teaspoon sea salt

½ teaspoon freshly ground white pepper

In a large bowl, combine the watermelon, blueberries, strawberries, mixed greens, and lemon zest; set aside in the refrigerator to chill for 10 minutes.

Whisk the remaining ingredients in a small bowl. Allow to chill in the refrigerator for 5 minutes.

Remove the salad and dressing from refrigerator. Drizzle the dressing over the salad; gently toss to combine. Add salt and pepper. Serve chilled.

CRANBERRY-QUINOA SALAD*

Serves 4

Salad:

1 cup quinoa

¼ cup dried cranberries

2 scallions, finely chopped

2 cups mixed greens, such as spinach and arugula

Dressing:

¼ cup cashews

⅛ cup pine nuts

2 teaspoons miso paste

¼ teaspoon agave nectar

3 tablespoons freshly squeezed lemon juice

2 garlic cloves, minced

1 tablespoon lemon zest

¼ teaspoon crushed red pepper

¼ teaspoon sea salt

¼ teaspoon freshly ground black pepper

Cook the quinoa according to the package directions.

While the quinoa cooks, combine all the dressing ingredients in a blender; process until smooth. Add ½ cup water if the dressing is too thick.

In a large serving bowl, combine the cooked quinoa, dried cranberries, scallions, and mixed greens; gently toss with the dressing to coat. Serve chilled.

RED RHUBARB QUINOA*

Serves 4

Salad:

2 heads butter lettuce

1½ cups red quinoa, cooked

1 cup shredded radishes

1 cup shredded purple cabbage

½ medium red onion, sliced

1 large carrot, shredded

1 large apple, peeled, cored, and sliced

1 pint cherry tomatoes

Dressing:

¼ cup honey

⅓ cup green tea, brewed

4 stalks rhubarb, sliced

½ shallot, sliced

⅓ cup apple cider vinegar

1 teaspoon spicy brown mustard

½ cup flaxseed oil

Garnish:

1 cup organic salsa

½ cup canned pumpkin

⅓ cup salted pistachios

Combine the lettuce, quinoa, radishes, cabbage, onion, carrot, apple, and tomatoes in a large salad bowl.

To make the dressing, combine the honey and tea in a medium saucepan and bring to a boil; add the rhubarb and shallot. Boil for 4 more minutes, stirring often. Reduce to a simmer; add the vinegar and cook for another 12 minutes, or until the liquid is reduced by half and the rhubarb is tender. Remove from the heat; set aside to cool.

Transfer the rhubarb mixture to a food processor with the mustard and flaxseed oil; pulse until smooth.

Serve atop the salad; garnish with a spoonful of salsa, pumpkin, and pistachios.

MAPLE SLAW SALAD*

Serves 4

Salad:

- 4 cups baby spinach
- ¼ cup baby arugula
- ½ small head Napa cabbage, shredded
- ½ small head red cabbage, shredded
- 2 large carrots, shredded
- 5 large radishes, shredded
- 1 cup fresh basil leaves
- ¼ cup finely chopped fresh parsley
- 1 teaspoon lemon zest
- ¼ cup pistachios

Dressing:

- 3 tablespoons olive oil
- ⅓ cup chopped shallots
- ⅔ cup apple cider vinegar
- 1 teaspoon chia seeds
- ¼ cup maple syrup
- 2 tablespoons freshly squeezed lemon juice

Combine the spinach, arugula, cabbages, carrots, radishes, basil, parsley, lemon zest, and pistachios in a large salad bowl; set aside.

To make the dressing, whisk the oil, shallots, vinegar, chia seeds, maple syrup, and lemon juice in a medium skillet; cook for 15 minutes. Remove from the heat; drizzle over the salad and serve.

BASIL-AVOCADO SALAD*

Serves 2

- 1 large fennel bulb, stalks and bulbs sliced into ½ inch pieces
- 2 cups baby arugula
- 1 ripe avocado, peeled, pitted, and sliced
- 1 large carrot, finely chopped
- Juice of 1 organic lemon
- 2 tablespoons extra-virgin olive oil
- ¼ teaspoon lemon zest
- 4 fresh basil leaves, finely chopped
- ¼ teaspoon sea salt

¼ teaspoon freshly ground
black pepper

2 tablespoons ground chia seeds

¼ cup cashews

Fill a large bowl with ice water.

Bring a large pot of salted water to a boil. Add the fennel and cook for 3 minutes. Drain the fennel and immediately submerge in the ice bath. Set aside for 3 minutes. Drain.

Transfer the fennel to a large serving bowl; pat dry. Add the arugula, avocado, and carrot.

Drizzle the salad with the lemon juice, oil, lemon zest, basil, salt, and pepper. Gently toss to coat.

Divide the salad between two serving dishes. Top with the chia seeds and cashews. Serve at room temperature.

PURPLE CABBAGE SALAD WITH EDAMAME, RAISINS, AND WALNUTS**

Serves 2

1½ cups frozen shelled edamame

2 cups thinly sliced purple cabbage

1 orange or red bell pepper, cored, seeded, and thinly sliced

1 cup finely diced pineapple

¼ cup golden raisins

¼ cup coarsely chopped walnuts

¼ cup chopped fresh mint

2 tablespoons freshly squeezed lime juice

2 tablespoons honey

¼ teaspoon chili-garlic sauce

Salt and freshly ground black pepper

Bring a small pot of water to a boil. Add the edamame and cook for 10 minutes. Drain, and refresh under cold water. Transfer to a large bowl; add the cabbage, bell pepper, pineapple, raisins, walnuts, mint, lime juice, honey, and chili-garlic sauce. Toss well and season with salt and pepper.

TOSSED ARUGULA SALAD

Serves 2

Salad:

½ cup shelled pumpkin seeds

1 teaspoon Bragg liquid
  amino acids

1 large red bell pepper, cut
  into ½-inch slices

1 large leek, cut into 1-inch pieces

3 tablespoons ghee

1 bunch of arugula

1 cup alfalfa sprouts

1 cup finely shredded daikon
  radish or jícama

1 cup watercress

Dressing:

2 tablespoons extra-virgin olive oil

1 tablespoon freshly
  squeezed lemon juice

1 teaspoon honey

1 teaspoon Dijon mustard

1 teaspoon dried thyme

1 teaspoon dried basil

½ teaspoon ground turmeric

¼ teaspoon paprika

Salt and freshly ground
  black pepper

Small handful of seedless
  raisins for garnish

Preheat the oven to 350°F. In a baking dish, spread the pumpkin seeds in a single layer and bake until golden brown, about 7 minutes. Remove from the oven, sprinkle with the Bragg's liquid amino acids (a substitute for soy sauce found at health food stores and grocery stores; it's nonfermented and salt-free, but it tastes the same), and stir well.

Increase the oven temperature to 400°F. Spread the bell pepper and leek on a baking sheet, drizzle with the ghee, and bake until soft, about 30 minutes.

In a large salad bowl, toss the pumpkin seeds, bell pepper, leek, arugula, alfalfa sprouts, daikon, and watercress.

In a mixing bowl, whisk the oil, lemon juice, honey, mustard, thyme, basil, turmeric, paprika, salt, and pepper.

Pour the dressing over the salad and toss. Garnish with raisins and serve.

GRILLED VEGETABLES WITH MISO SAUCE**

Serves 2

Vegetables:

¼ red kuri or green kabocha squash, seeded and cut into ½-inch-thick slices

1 small red onion, sliced

2 teaspoons sesame oil

Organic cooking spray

1 large bok choy, leaves separated

Miso Sauce:

1 tablespoon miso paste

1 garlic clove, minced

½ teaspoon light brown sugar

¼ cup water

1 teaspoon sesame oil

½ teaspoon rice vinegar

2 scallions, chopped (about ¼ cup)

1 tablespoon toasted sesame seeds

To make the vegetables, brush the squash and onion slices with the oil. Spray a grill with cooking spray, and lay the squash slices on the grill. Close, and cook on medium-high heat for 10 minutes, or until the squash is tender; transfer to a plate. Place the onion on the grill; cook for 4 to 5 minutes, until crisp-tender, and transfer to a plate. Place the bok choy on the grill; cook for 3 to 4 minutes, until wilted and crisp-tender, and transfer to a plate.

Meanwhile, to make the miso sauce, combine the miso paste, garlic, brown sugar, and water in a small saucepan. Bring to a simmer over medium heat. Cook for 2 minutes, or until the miso dissolves and begins to bloom. Remove from the heat; stir in the oil and vinegar. Fold in the scallions and sesame seeds.

Serve the grilled vegetables drizzled with the miso sauce, or serve the miso sauce on the side.

POTATO-BASIL PUREE

Serves 4 or 5

2 cups fresh basil leaves,
   lightly packed

2 pounds large Yukon gold or
   white boiling potatoes,
   boiled and quartered

1 cup half-and-half

¾ cup freshly grated Parmesan
   cheese plus more for serving

2 teaspoons kosher salt
   plus more to taste

1 teaspoon freshly ground black
   pepper plus more to taste

Bring a large pot of salted water to a boil and fill a bowl with ice water. Add the basil to the boiling water and cook for exactly 15 seconds. Remove the basil with a slotted spoon and immediately plunge the leaves into the ice water to set the bright green color. Drain and set aside.

Add the potatoes to the same pot of boiling water and return to a boil. Cook for 20 to 25 minutes, until very tender. Drain well, return to the pot, and steam over low heat until any remaining water evaporates.

In a small saucepan over medium heat, combine the half-and-half and Parmesan and heat until the cream simmers. Place the basil in a food processor fitted with the steel blade and puree. Add the hot cream mixture and process until smooth.

With a hand mixer, beat the hot potatoes in the pot until they are broken up. Slowly add the hot basil cream, salt, and pepper and beat until smooth. If the potatoes need to be reheated, cover and cook over low heat for a few minutes. Pour into a serving bowl, sprinkle with more Parmesan, and season to taste. Serve hot.

FLAXSEED PESTO ON SPAGHETTI SQUASH†

Serves 6

2 whole spaghetti squash

1 cup fresh basil leaves, washed and patted dry, plus more for garnish

1 cup fresh cilantro leaves, washed and patted dry, plus more garnish

2 garlic cloves, chopped

½ cup golden flaxseed

1 cup extra-virgin olive oil

1 cup freshly grated Parmesan cheese or nutritional yeast

¼ cup freshly grated Romano cheese

½ teaspoon salt

½ teaspoon freshly ground black pepper

Preheat the oven to 400°F.

Place the spaghetti squash in a baking dish. Pierce in several places with a fork. Place in the oven and bake for about 1 hour.

Combine the basil, cilantro, garlic, and flaxseed in the bowl of a food processor or blender and chop.

Leave the motor running and add the oil in a slow, steady stream.

Shut off the motor; add the cheeses, salt, and pepper. Process or blend briefly to combine, then scrape out into a bowl and cover until ready to use.

When the squash is cooked through (test with a fork or knife; it should pierce easily), remove from the oven. Let cool for a few minutes before handling. Cut the squash in half and scoop out the seeds with a spoon. With a fork, scrape out the "spaghetti" into a large pasta bowl. Cover to keep warm until ready to serve.

Spoon the pesto over the "spaghetti." Garnish with chopped fresh cilantro and a few fresh basil leaves. Serve.

KALE AND CRANBERRY SALAD

Serves 4

1 bunch kale, chopped into
   bite-size pieces

¼ cup cranberries

1 carrot, shredded

½ cucumber, thinly sliced

1 medium tomato, diced

2 or 3 small red radishes,
   finely chopped

1 tablespoon sunflower seeds

2 tablespoons extra-virgin olive oil

1 teaspoon lemon juice

Combine all the ingredients, toss, and serve.

PUMPKIN SOUP

Serves 4

1 large onion, diced

2 tablespoons olive oil

2 to 3 garlic cloves

2 teaspoons minced fresh ginger

2 to 4 carrots, diced

1½ tablespoons curry powder

½ teaspoon cayenne pepper

½ teaspoon ground cinnamon

¼ teaspoon ground nutmeg

4 cups chicken or vegetable broth

1 large sweet potato,
   baked with skin

1 medium pumpkin, baked
   and cut into chunks

Greek yogurt for garnish

Toss the onion with the oil, garlic, ginger, and carrots. Transfer to a
heated large pot and sauté for 2 to 4 minutes, until the onion is cara-
melized. Add the curry powder, cayenne, cinnamon, nutmeg, and
broth. Bring to a boil, then reduce the heat, cover, and simmer for 10
to 15 minutes. Peel and cut the sweet potato into chunks. Add to the
broth with the pumpkin. Cook for 3 to 5 minutes. Puree the soup
in a food processor or blender in batches. Return to the pot, simmer,
and add water to create a thinner consistency, if desired. Season to
taste. Ladle into bowls and garnish with plain Greek yogurt.

BUTTERNUT SQUASH SOUP‡

Serves 6

1 tablespoon olive oil

5 ounces pancetta, cut
   into small dice

1 yellow onion, chopped

1 teaspoon peeled and
   minced apple

2 garlic cloves, minced

1 sprig fresh sage

1¼ cups low-sodium chicken broth

1 (32-ounce) jar butternut
   squash puree

Salt

Freshly ground white pepper

¼ cup heavy cream

Lightly whipped cream for garnish

¼ cup hazelnuts, toasted
   and chopped

Heat the oil in a large pot over medium-low heat. Add the pancetta
and cook, stirring occasionally, until lightly crisp, 5 to 7 minutes.
Transfer to a paper towel–lined plate; reserve the oil in the pot.

Add the onion and apple to the pot; cook, stirring occasionally,
until tender, 8 to 10 minutes. Add the garlic and sage sprig; cook,
stirring, for 1 minute. Add the broth and squash puree; simmer for
10 to 15 minutes. Remove the sage sprig and discard. Reduce the
heat to low; simmer for a few minutes. Add salt and pepper. Simmer
for 3 minutes. Remove from the heat. Using an immersion blender,
puree the soup until smooth. Whisk in the heavy cream. Ladle into
warmed bowls; garnish with the pancetta, a dollop of whipped
cream, and the hazelnuts.

ASPARAGUS SOUP

Serves 4

4 cups finely chopped asparagus

2 cups finely chopped celery

6 cups chicken or vegetable broth

6 tablespoons butter or ghee

¼ teaspoon freshly ground
    black pepper

¼ teaspoon ground nutmeg

¼ cup rice flour

1 cup heavy cream

Steam the asparagus and celery for 5 minutes in a large pot, then puree the asparagus and celery in a blender. Return to the pot, add the broth, butter, pepper, and nutmeg, and cook for 20 minutes on medium heat. Add the flour and cream to thicken. Reduce the heat to medium-low. Serve warm.

SPRING CARROT SOUP

Serves 4

1 tablespoon extra-virgin olive
    oil or clarified butter

2 garlic cloves, minced

1 large yellow onion, chopped

3 cups vegetable broth or water

1¼ pounds carrots, cut
    into 1-inch pieces

Juice of ½ lemon

Fine-grain sea salt

Heat the oil in a large pot over medium heat. Add the garlic and onion and sauté for a few minutes, or until the onion starts to get translucent. Add the broth and carrots. Lower the heat and simmer for 20 to 30 minutes, until the carrots are tender—longer if your carrot pieces ended up larger (but try not to overcook). Remove from the heat and let cool for a few minutes.

Puree with an immersion blender, then stir in the lemon juice. Season with salt and serve.

BRAISED CHICKEN WITH CILANTRO-REDUCTION SAUCE

Serves 4

2 tablespoons ghee

4 boneless, skinless chicken breasts

Salt and freshly ground
    black pepper

1 cup organic chicken or
    vegetable broth

1 bunch of fresh cilantro

2 cups filtered water

1 teaspoon grated fresh ginger

1 teaspoon ground fennel seeds

¼ teaspoon ground turmeric

½ teaspoon salt-free seasoning
    mixture (dried herbs and
    spices) of your choice

½ teaspoon maple syrup

10 fresh mint leaves, chopped

1 to 2 tablespoons chickpea flour

Preheat the oven to 350°F.

Grease a baking dish with 1 tablespoon of the ghee. Place the chicken breasts in the dish and coat them with the ghee. Season with salt and pepper. Pour in the broth. Bake until the chicken is fully cooked, about 25 minutes.

While the chicken is cooking, combine the cilantro and 1 cup of the water in a blender or food processor. Blend or process until the mixture is smooth.

Heat the remaining 1 tablespoon ghee in a large saucepan over medium heat. Add the ginger and sauté for 2 minutes. Add the fennel seeds and sauté for 1 minute more. Stir in the turmeric, seasoning mixture, maple syrup, mint, cilantro puree, and the remaining 1 cup water. Simmer until reduced by half, about 20 minutes. Whisk in the chickpea flour and continue cooking, stirring continuously, until the sauce thickens, 2 to 3 minutes. Season to taste with salt and pepper.

To serve, arrange the chicken breasts on plates and pour the sauce over them.

LEMON-ROASTED ASPARAGUS

Serves 6

¼ cup olive oil

Juice of 1 lemon

2 pounds asparagus, trimmed

½ head cabbage, cored and
   cut into 4 strips

¼ cup Bragg liquid amino acids

2 tablespoons light brown sugar

2 tablespoons dried cherries

1 tablespoon minced fresh ginger

2 oranges, peeled and sectioned

2 tablespoons chopped scallions

Preheat the oven to 400°F.

Combine the oil and lemon juice in a bowl. Immerse the asparagus
and cabbage, coating completely. Place the asparagus and cabbage
on a baking sheet, spreading evenly. Roast for 5 minutes, until crisp-
tender. Turn the vegetables over. Roast for another 5 to 10 minutes,
until desired tenderness.

Combine the amino acids, sugar, cherries, and ginger in a bowl; stir
well. Add the orange sections.

Place the asparagus and cabbage on a platter. Add the orange
mixture to the top. Garnish with the scallions.

SPICED BALSAMIC BEET COMPOTE

Serves 6

½ cup golden raisins

2 large beets, peeled and finely
    diced (about 3 cups)

2 tablespoons olive oil

½ teaspoon garam masala
    or curry powder

2 shallots, halved and thinly
    sliced (about ½ cup)

2 tablespoons balsamic vinegar

1 teaspoon salt

Cover the raisins with boiling water, and let stand for 30 minutes. Drain.

Meanwhile, cook the beets in a large pot of boiling water for 10 minutes, or until just tender. Drain, and set aside.

Heat the oil in a large skillet over medium heat. Add the garam masala, and cook for 20 seconds, or until fragrant. Add the shallots, and sauté for 2 minutes. Stir in the beets, raisins, vinegar, salt, and ½ cup of water. Cover, and simmer for 20 minutes, or until the compote is thickened. Let cool.

STEWED APPLES WITH CLOVES AND CINNAMON

Serves 2

2 apples, peeled, cored, and sliced

5 dried apricots, soaked in hot water for 20 minutes

4 Medjool dates, pitted and cut in half

2 cups filtered water

1 tablespoon maple syrup

1 tablespoon grated fresh ginger

¼ teaspoon ground cardamom

¼ teaspoon ground cinnamon

1 teaspoon whole cloves

Combine the apples, apricots, dates, water, maple syrup, ginger, cardamom, cinnamon, and cloves in a medium saucepan and bring to a boil over high heat. Reduce the heat to medium-low and cover. Simmer for 5 minutes.

Transfer one third of the contents (including the juice) to a blender or a food processor and mix until pureed. Stir the puree back into the pan and serve warm.

MINT TEA

Serves 2

2 cups filtered water

12 fresh mint leaves, or 1 organic peppermint tea bag

In a saucepan, bring the water to a boil. Reduce the heat to a simmer and stir in the mint leaves.

Pour the water and mint into a teapot and let brew for 10 minutes.

Strain the tea and serve hot. Alternatively, serve cold by refrigerating the strained tea and then pouring over ice.

HOT QUINOA CEREAL WITH WARM SPICED MILK

Serves 2

1 cup filtered water	¼ teaspoon ground ginger
½ cup quinoa	Pinch of ground cinnamon
1 cup organic soy milk	2 tablespoons honey

Bring the water and quinoa to a boil in a small saucepan over high heat. Lower the heat and simmer, stirring frequently, until the quinoa is tender and the mixture thickens, about 20 minutes. Add more water if necessary.

When the quinoa is nearly done, combine the soy milk, ginger, and cinnamon in a separate saucepan. Warm the mixture over low heat.

Divide the quinoa into two servings. Pour the warm spiced soy milk over each serving and drizzle with honey.

CILANTRO PESTO SAUCE

Makes 1½ cups

2 tablespoons pine nuts	2 teaspoons lemon juice
1 cup fresh cilantro leaves	2 tablespoons water
3 tablespoons extra-virgin olive oil	Salt and freshly ground
3 tablespoons organic plain yogurt	black pepper

Preheat the oven to 350°F.

On a baking sheet, spread the pine nuts in a single layer and bake, stirring occasionally, until toasted to a golden brown, about 10 minutes. Transfer to a plate and let cool.

In a blender or food processor, combine the toasted pine nuts, cilantro, oil, yogurt, lemon juice, and water. Blend or process until the mixture forms a thick, smooth paste. Season to taste with salt and pepper.

BLACK BEAN TACOS WITH MANGO SALSA

Serves 1

Salsa:

1 tablespoon whole cumin seeds

1 ripe mango, peeled and chopped

½ teaspoon finely chopped
  green chili

½ teaspoon crushed garlic

1 teaspoon paprika

1 tablespoon lime juice

1 tablespoon chopped fresh parsley

Tacos:

2 small or medium organic
  corn tortillas

½ cup canned organic black beans

1 medium tomato, chopped

1 small red bell pepper, diced

½ ripe avocado, diced

¼ cup chopped fresh cilantro

To prepare the salsa, roast the cumin seeds in a small dry sauté pan over low heat until fragrant, 1 to 2 minutes. Stir all its ingredients in a mixing bowl. Cover and refrigerate until serving time.

To assemble, place the tortillas on a plate. On top of each tortilla neatly spread the beans, tomato, bell pepper, avocado, and cilantro. Add the salsa if desired.

Optional: For more protein, add diced chicken from an organic, roasted chicken.

Recipe Credits

* Based on a recipe by Amie Valpone at TheHealthyApple.com.

** Based on a recipe published by VegetarianTimes.com.

† Based on a recipe by Ed Bauman, MEd, PhD, BaumanCollege.com.

‡ Based on a recipe by the Williams-Sonoma Kitchen.

Appendix B: Glossary of Ayurvedic Terms

agni: fire, particularly the digestive fire

ama: residual impurities and toxic material caused by poor digestion

amla: sour taste

ananda: bliss

anna: food

annavaha srotas: digestive system

apas: the element of water

artava: menstrual fluid

artavavaha srotas: menstrual system

artha: the goal of attaining wealth, resources, or possessions

asana: a yoga pose

atman: inner self

Ayurveda: the spiritual science of life (a branch of Vedas)

bahya marga: outer disease pathway (skin and blood)

bala: bodily strength

bhakti yoga: yoga of devotion

bhuta: element

bhutagni: digestive fire governing an element

brahmacharya: control of sexual energy

darshana: system of philosophy

dharana: concentration, attention

dharma: goal, principle, law of one's nature

dhatu: one of the body's seven basic components, synonymous with "tissue" in Western medicine

dhatvagni: agni in the tissues

dhyana: meditation, contemplation

dinacharya: daily regimen

gati: movement

ghee: clarified butter

gunas: attributes, fundamental qualities of nature

guru: quality of heaviness; spiritual teacher

hatha yoga: yoga of physical postures

hridaya: heart

japa: repetition of mantras

jatharagni: digestive fire

jiva: individual soul

jnana yoga: yoga of knowledge

jyotish: Vedic astrology

kala: nutritional membrane for the tissues

kama: desire

kapha: the dosha that governs bodily structure

karma: bondage to action, the cause of rebirth

karma yoga: yoga of service

kashaya: astringent taste

katu: pungent or spicy taste

kshatriya: warrior

Kundalini: dormant serpent energy

laghu: lightness

madhyama marga: middle disease pathway (deep tissue)

majja: bone marrow and nerve tissue

mala: waste material of the body

mamsa: muscle

manas: mind as principle of thought

mantra: words of power, sacred sounds

marga: pathway of the body

marma: vital points on the body

maya: illusion; cosmic creative power

medas: fat

moksha: liberation

mutra: urine

mutravaha srotas: urinary system

nadi: Ayurvedic name for pulse

nasya: nasal administration of therapies

nyaya: one of the six Indian systems of philosophy

ojas: primary energy reserve of the body and mind; the pure outcome of perfect digestion and metabolism

panchakarma: five cleansing actions of vomiting, purgation, enemas, bloodletting, and nasal medications

pariksha: examination or diagnosis

pitta: the dosha that governs metabolism

prabhava: special action of herbs

prajñaparadha: mistaken intellect

prakriti: primal nature, natural state, constitution

prana: life force, breath, subtle form of the life force, inward moving of the five breaths or life force in the head

Pranayama: controlled, breathing exercises

pratyahara: control of senses and mind

purisha: feces

purishavaha srotas: excretory system

purusha: the original spirit, inner self

rajas: the principle of energy among the three qualities of nature (gunas)

rajasic: having the nature of rajas

rakta: blood

raktavaha srotas: circulatory system (hemoglobin portion)

rasa: plasma; taste

rasayana: rejuvenation

ritucharya: seasonal regimen

roga: disease

sattva: the higher principle of harmony of the three qualities of nature (gunas)

sattvic: having the nature of sattva

satya: truth

satya buddhi: ascertainment of truth

shakti: power, energy of consciousness

shamana: palliation therapy

shita: cool

shiva: pure being or pure consciousness

shodhana: purification therapy

shukra: reproductive fluid

shukravaha srotas: reproductive system

siddhi: psychic power

snehana: oil massage therapy

soma: bliss or pleasure principle at work behind the mind and senses

sparshana: touch, palpation

srotas: the different channel systems or physiological systems

Sushruta: ancient Ayurvedic author

sutra: axiom used in Vedic teaching

swastha: health

swasthavritta: regimen promoting health

swasthya: state of being healthy

swedana: steam or sweating therapy

tail: medicated oil

tamas: the lower principle of inertia of the three qualities of nature (gunas)

tamasic: having the nature of tamas

tanmatra: five prime sensory principles (sound, touch, sight, taste, and smell) behind organs and elements

tantra: medieval yoga traditions emphasizing use of techniques and rituals

tapas: discipline, self-discipline

tejas: fire on a vital level

tikta: bitter taste

udana vayu: upward moving of the five breaths

upanishads: ancient Vedantic teachings of India

ushna: hot

Vagbhatta: ancient Ayurvedic author

Vaidya: Ayurvedic doctor

vaisheshika: one of the six systems of Indian philosophy

vajikarana: aphrodisiac

vata: the dosha that governs all movement in the body

vayas: life span

vayu: another name for vata

vedanta: culmination of the Vedas in the philosophy of self-realization

Vedas: ancient books of knowledge presenting the spiritual science of awareness

vijñana: intelligence

vikriti: disease state, diversification or deviation from nature

vikriti pariksha: examination of disease

vipaka: post-digestive effect of herbs

virya: energetic effect of herbs as heating or cooling

vishuddha chakra: throat chakra

vyana vayu: outward moving of the five breaths

yama: right attitudes in yoga practice

yoga: psychophysical practices aimed at self-knowledge

yoga sutras: classical textbook of yoga

Acknowledgments

This book has provided me a precious opportunity to look back and reflect upon my own journey—a journey that started in rural India and after several stops in many continents, found its perfect landing in America. Along my path, countless hands, guides, and mentors have shared their love and wisdom with me and I express my sincere gratitude to all of them.

First and foremost, I thank my wife, Manisha, who accepted me "as is" and quietly changed the very fabric of my life to make it abundant, beautiful, and happy. I thank her for all her support in every area of my life and the two blessings we have together, our children, Manas and Sanika. They were so kind, flexible, and loving that they never complained when they traveled with us to so many countries and attended many different schools. Their unconditional love is my greatest gift.

A heartfelt thanks goes to Marci Shimoff (bestselling author of *Happy for No Reason*), who discovered the author in me and made the project a virtual reality. She is the one who first introduced me to my agent, Bonnie Solow, and later to Kristin Loberg, who together brought this book to life.

I am forever grateful to His Holiness Maharishi Mahesh Yogi, the founder of the Transcendental Meditation movement, who not only gave me the insights on higher states of consciousness, but also helped me understand the true value of Vedic science and its modern-day application.

This book would not have been possible without the extraordinary efforts of Kristin Loberg, who is a gifted writer, a brilliant mind, and a loving friend. She worked tirelessly on *The Hot Belly Diet* with the big belly of an expectant mother. I respect her dedication and professional ethics.

A heartfelt thank-you to the publishing team at Atria, who was willing to take a leap of faith and has been such a joy to work with. A special thanks goes out to Judith Curr, Sarah Durand, and Daniella Wexler; it's truly an honor and a privilege to work with you. Sarah, your brilliant editorial eye and vision for the book helped me transform the manuscript into a beautiful, polished product. Thanks for your leadership. Thank you also to Elaine Broeder, Lisa Sciambra, and Paul Olsewski in publicity; Hillary Tisman in marketing; Jeanne Lee, art director; and Lisa Keim, foreign rights director. Such an amazing, dedicated group of talented people.

I would like to convey my deepest gratitude to Dr. Deepak Chopra, for his inspiration, wisdom, and vision. He supported the whole project from the very beginning and he has been a magnificent mentor and a wonderful friend. He is a master at what he does and I feel blessed to have learned from the very best.

I fondly remember and thank the late Dr. David Simon (the cofounder of The Chopra Center) for his friendship and vision. He, along with Deepak, was the true pioneer of mind-body medicine that laid a solid foundation for modern-day Ayurveda.

To Bonnie Solow, my literary agent and a dear friend, who guided us on this wonderful project with steady support and encouragement. I deeply admire your attention to detail, unwavering positive attitude, incredible patience, and willingness to work with first-time authors like me.

I also want to express my sincere gratitude to the many trailblazers, like Tony Robbins and Drs. Wayne Dyer, Mehmet Oz, Eckhart Tolle, Dean Ornish, Andrew Weil, and David Frawley, who have inspired millions to lead a healthy and happy life.

I deeply appreciate The Chopra Center physicians Sheila Patel, Tim Brieske, and Valencia Porter, and all the staff members who make The Chopra Center a magical healing place.

Dr. Tom Yarema has been a true friend who has not only helped my immigration process, but also helped me refine my teaching and clinical skills. We are like long-lost brothers from two different continents who continue to work and grow together.

I sincerely miss my late friend Daniel Rhoda, who always believed in me and led me on my reincarnation to create Zrii.

I want to thank my dear friend Bill Farley (owner and CEO of Zrii), who is a remarkable visionary and was always supportive and firm in his belief about my talent and skill sets. I am thankful for the opportunity to formulate products for Zrii.

To my inspiring colleagues at Maharishi University of Management: Drs. Keith Wallace, Robert Schneider, Stuart Rothenberg, Nancy Lonsdorf, John Hagelin, and Paul Morehead. You are the beacons of Vedic wisdom and its integrative approach.

I also would like to thank my Ayurvedic colleagues: Drs. Vasant Lad, Jay Apte, Vivek Shanbhag, Annambhotala Shekhar, Jayarajan, Subhash Ranade, Avinash Lele, and P. H. Kulkarni, for your tireless pursuit to make Ayurveda a household name in the West.

A special thanks to Ramesh Vangal from Kerala Ayurveda for his positive energy and steadfast support.

I am deeply grateful for and forever blessed with my lovely family, my parents, my in-laws, my brother, Vilas, and his family, my sister and her family, and my brother-in-law, Rajendra, and his family. I respect and appreciate your loving support.

My staff at Ayurvedic Healing has been a solid rock to anchor all my travels and changing schedules. Thanks for your patience and smiling faces.

Last, but not least, I want to thank all of my clients and students throughout the years. I have gained so much because you have allowed me into your lives and have shared with me your stories, challenges, and personal journeys. You should know you hold a very special place in my heart.

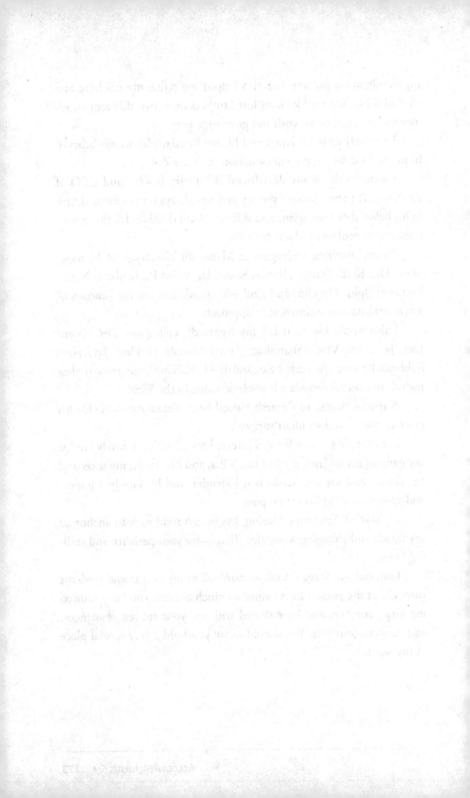

Resources

The following is a partial list of resources to check out in living by the Hot Diet Belly principles. You can also go to www.hotbellydiet.com for additional resources and updated lists.

Ayurvedic Healing
Dr. Suhas Kshirsagar (Ayu, MD, India)
Dr. Manisha Kshirsagar (Ayu, BAMS, India)
3121 Park Ave., Suite D
Soquel, CA 95073
Tel. 831-462-3776
www.AyurvedicHealing.Net

Center for Wellness & Integrative Medicine
Dr. Tom Yarema, MD
3121 Park Ave., Suite D
Soquel, CA 95073
Tel. 831-462-3776
drtomyarema.com

The Chopra Center for Wellbeing
Deepak Chopra, MD
2013 Costa Del Mar Rd.
Carlsbad, CA 92009
Tel. 760-494-1639
www.chopra.com

Arizona Center for Integrative Medicine
Andrew Weil, MD
P.O. Box 245153
Tucson, AZ 85724
Tel. 520-626-6417
www.integrativemedicine.arizona.edu

Maharishi Ayurveda Products
1680 Highway 1 North
Suite 2200
Fairfield, Iowa 52556
Tel. 800-255-8332
www.mapi.com

David Frawley and Yogini Shambhavi
American Institute of Vedic Studies
P.O. Box 8357
Santa Fe, NM 87504-8357
Tel. 505-983-9385
www.vedanet.com

The Ayurvedic Institute and Wellness Center
Dr. Vasant Lad, BAMS, MAS
11311 Menaul Blvd. NE
Albuquerque, NM 87112
Tel. 505-291-9698
www.ayurveda.com

The Raj
1734 Jasmine Ave.
Vedic City, Fairfield, IA 52556
Tel. 800-864-8714
www.theraj.com

Dean Ornish, MD
Preventive Medicine Research Institute
900 Bridgeway
Sausalito, CA 94965
Tel. 415-332-2525

Kerala Ayurveda Academy
46500 Fremont Blvd, Suite 702
Fremont, CA 94538
Tel. 888-275-9103
www.ayurvedaacademy.com

Yoga Directory By State
www.self-realization.com/yogadirectory.htm

Banyan Botanicals
6705 Eagle Rock Ave. NE,
Albuquerque, NM 87113
Tel. 800-953-6424
www.banyanbotanicals.com

Index

A

activity, 56, 82
  see also exercise
addictions, 220–21
age, 230
aging, 2, 12
  agni and, 40
agni, *see* digestive fire
alcohol, 94, 121, 150
Allen, Woody, 225
Almond, Strawberry, and Arugula
  Salad, 242–43
ama, 32–36, 40–43, 59, 64, 69, 174,
  193
  diagnosing, 52–53
  food combinations and, 124
  gluten and, 41
  inflammation and, 40
  properties of, 33
  signs of, 44
amalaki, 90
American Cancer Society, 155
American Diabetes Association, 62
American Dietetic Association
  (ADA), 61
American Journal of Epidemiology,
  155
American Society for Nutrition, 70
appetite, 59
  see also hunger
Apples, Stewed, with Cloves and
  Cinnamon, 260

Archives of Internal Medicine, 65
artificial sweeteners, 93–94
arugula:
  Strawberry, Almond, and Arugula
    Salad, 242–43
  Tossed Arugula Salad, 250–51
asparagus:
  Asparagus Soup, 256
  Lemon-Roasted Asparagus, 258
ATP, 153
Avocado-Basil Salad, 248–49
Ayurveda, 1–4, 10–14, 16–18,
  20, 23, 24, 27, 28, 40, 81,
  172, 174, 184, 185, 190,
  199–200
  body types in, *see* doshas
  cycles in, 54–55
  defining, 10
  exercise and, 157–58
  glossary of terms used in,
    265–70
  mind and body in, 71–72
  nutrition in, 115–17
  obesity as viewed in, 151
  pairings in, 158
  self-referral and, 11, 194
  Western medicine and, 16–17,
    172
Ayurvedic supplements, 89
  trikatu, 69, 91–92
  triphala, 69, 89–91
ayus (life), 27–28

mood and, 65
net, 67
processed, cutting, 92–93
satisfaction from, 70
sensitivity to, 68–69, 104, 107
simple, 64–65
weight and, 64, 65–66
see also grains
Carrot Soup, Spring, 256
castor oil cleanse, 64, 86–89, 113, 227
Centers for Disease Control and Prevention (CDC), 147
Cereal, Hot Quinoa, with Warm Spiced Milk, 261
Charaka, 24, 141, 142–43, 157
Chicken, Braised, with Cilantro-Reduction Sauce, 257
chewing, 112–13
cholesterol, 58, 66–67, 128, 147, 150, 155
cilantro:
　Braised Chicken with Cilantro-Reduction Sauce, 257
　Cilantro Pesto Sauce, 261–62
　Flaxseed Pesto on Spaghetti Squash, 253
circadian rhythm, 54–57, 111
Citrusy Kale Salad with Blueberries and Pumpkin Seeds, 239
Classic Sweet Lassi, 236
clock, internal, 54–57, 111
Coconut-Cucumber Smoothie, 234
comfort foods, 70
cranberry:
　Cranberry-Quinoa Salad, 246
　Kale and Cranberry Salad, 254
cravings, 22, 61, 62, 85, 94, 101, 143, 167
　for carbohydrates, 64
Cucumber-Coconut Smoothie, 234

Curry, Butternut Squash and Spinach, 242

D
dairy, 58, 93, 121
　food combinations and, 124–25
deepana, 59
dessert, 109
dhatus, 173–74, 192
diabetes, 58, 61, 62, 68, 147–49, 156, 190
diet foods, 93
digestive fire (agni), 2, 10, 17, 18, 20, 24, 28–36, 38–39, 41–42, 44, 48, 121
　aging and, 40
　calories and, 59
　and fasting between meals, 112
　four main states of, 32
　gluten and, 41
　healthy, signs of, 33
　kapha and, 75
　khichadi and, 57
　liquids and, 76–77, 119, 125
　multiple meals and, 59
　obesity and, 151
　Phase 1 and, 85
　pitta and, 75
　properties of, 33
　strong, four components of, 18–19
　tissues and, 173
　vata and, 75
　walking and, 159
　weak, test of, 34
digestive sludge, 19, 31, 33, 36, 85
　see also ama
digestive system, 2, 18, 25–27, 32, 36, 59, 174, 175–78, 193
　bacteria in, 178–84
　brain and, 177–78
　castor oil cleanse and, 86–89

Hot Quinoa Cereal with Warm
Spiced Milk, 261
Human Microbiome Project (HMP),
178
humors, 72
hunger, 18, 22, 27, 42, 59–61, 64,
111–12, 112, 177, 226
blood sugar and, 112
hunger meter test, 78–79, 103

I

immune system, 63, 165, 167, 179,
180, 182, 185
indigestion, 171
industrialized foods, 191, 193
inflammation, 36–39, 150, 177, 179
ama and, 40
circadian rhythms and, 55
ingredients and products:
allowable, 97–99
to remove, 95–96
Institute for Clinical and
Experimental Medicine, 62
insulin, 61, 69, 156
insulin resistance, 68, 188
internal clock, 54–57, 111
intestinal sludge, 19, 31, 33, 36, 85
see also ama
irritability, 229–30

J

Journal of Nutrition, 65, 66, 70
journals, 213
juicing, 58

K

Kahleova, Hana, 62
kale:
Citrusy Kale Salad with
Blueberries and Pumpkin
Seeds, 239
Kale and Cranberry Salad, 254

Kale and Mandarin Salad, 237
Kale Tabbouleh, 241
Tuscan Kale, 240
kapha, 16, 30, 36, 39, 72, 73, 112,
121, 171, 186
characteristics of, 75
digestive fire and, 75
disease stages and, 185, 188, 191
exercise and, 144, 158, 160, 161
general dietary tips for, 127
unbalanced, 187
walking and, 158
kayakalpa, 45
khichadi, 19, 57–58, 66, 70, 104, 227
Gourmet Khichadi, 235
Midday Khichadi, 106–8, 234
Suppertime Khichadi, 108–9,
235
kitchen products and ingredients:
allowable, 97–99
to remove, 95–96

L

Lactobacillus acidophilus, 179
lassi, 108
Classic Sweet Lassi, 236
Salty (Digestive) Lassi, 236
lemon:
Lemon-Roasted Asparagus, 258
Lemon Squash Salad, 244–45
leptin, 155
life (ayus), 27–28
life's bigger picture, 219–20
lifestyle, 199–200
liquids, 18, 102
agni and, 76–77, 119, 125
to avoid, 78
bottled water, 78
cold and carbonated, 125
green tea drink, 102, 109
and fasting for a day, 87
hot, 76–78, 109, 207

morning drink, 119–20
sugary beverages, 94
liver, 26, 167, 181–82
castor oil and, 86
love, 224
lunch, 19, 45, 56–57, 62–63, 101, 215
khichadi and, 57
in Phase 2, 105, 107–8
regular schedule for, 111
timing of, 129
lymph, 165

M

Maharishi Mahesh Yogi, 14
malas, 192
Mandarin and Kale Salad, 237
Mango Salsa, Black Bean Tacos with, 262
Maple Slaw Salad, 248
massage, self-oil, 213–14
Mayo Clinic, 64
meals:
breakfast, 20, 56, 57, 62–63
dinner, see dinner
eating less during, 218
eating out, 134–35, 229
giving thanks before, 214–15
lunch, see lunch
mindfulness during, 110–13, 213
missing, 61
multiple, 59–63
passive entertainment while eating, 213
portions in, 78
regular schedule for, 111
resting after, 113
timing of, 129
walking after, 109–10, 113, 158, 159
meat, 58, 93, 101, 121, 128
medications, 92, 228
meditation, 209–11
memory, 65, 154

metabolic syndrome, 58
metabolism, 2, 18, 19, 32, 42, 59, 60, 69, 165, 170, 179
castor oil cleanse and, 86
daily drink and, 102
exercise and, 153
fasting and, 87
inflammation and, 38
multiple meals and, 61
warm water and, 77
see also digestive fire
metabolomics, 151–52
microwave ovens, 123–24
Midday Khichadi, 106–8, 234
milk, 124, 125
mind, 194–95
body and, 71–72, 184–85
mindful moderation, 121–23
mindfulness while eating, 110–13, 213
minerals, 70
Mint Tea, 260
mitochondria, 153
mood, 58, 62
carbohydrates and, 65
morning drink, 119–20
multitasking, 216

N

National Institutes of Health (NIH), 149, 178
nature, 168, 169, 200, 218–19
nervous system, 166, 167
New York Academy of Sciences, 62
nutrition, 25–26, 116
Ayurvedic, 115–17
taste and, 117, 118

O

ojas, 42, 43, 174
and mindfulness while eating, 110–13
signs of, 44